Praise for *Of Tears and Triumphs*

"The combination of excellent medical care, strong religious belief and supportive friends produced a joyful survivor, as this upbeat, celebratory and helpful guide attests."
—*Publishers Weekly*

"This is a pragmatic and dramatic book about survival, a war memorial that can and should be read not only by those who are ill but by those loved ones, family and friends who are touched by that illness."
—*Chicago Tribune*

"The words of Georgia and Bud breathe love, wisdom, and hope. *Of Tears and Triumphs* provides a rich source of understanding and realistic advice for all who face cancer."
—Irving I. Rimer
Vice President for Public Information
American Cancer Society

"Bud and Georgia are brave, admirable people, and all of us can benefit from what they have to tell us."
—Bob Greene
Syndicated Columnist

"This book is a true inspiration to us all. But more than anything else, this story is one of hope . . . of love, friends, family, and yes, of life itself."
—LaSalle D. Leffall, Jr., M.D.
Professor and Chairman
Department of Surgery
Howard University Hospital

Nov. 2004

Of Tears and Triumphs

GEORGIA AND BUD PHOTOPULOS

*With prayers
and Best Wishes —*

Georgia & Bud

CONGDON & WEED, INC.
Chicago

Library of Congress Cataloging-in-Publication Data

Photopulos, Georgia.
    Of tears and triumphs / Georgia and Bud Photopulos ;
foreword by LaSalle D. Leffall, Jr.
        p.   cm.
    ISBN 0-86553-197-8 (cloth)
        0-86553-218-4 (paper)
    1. Photopulos, Georgia—Health.   2. Photopulos,
Bud.   3. Breast—Cancer—Patients—United States—
Biography.   4. Cancer—Psychological aspects.
I. Photopulos, Bud.   II. Title.
RC280.B8P487   1988
362.1'9699449'00—dc19
[B]   88-19186
                                                          CIP

Copyright © 1988 by Bud and Georgia Photopulos
Library of Congress Catalog Card Number: 88-19186
International Standard Book Number:
        0-86553-197-8 (cloth)
        0-8092-0197-8Z (Contemporary Books, Inc.)
        0-86553-218-4 (paper)
        0-8092-0218-4Z (Contemporary Books, Inc.)
Published by Congdon & Weed, Inc.
A subsidiary of Contemporary Books, Inc.
Distributed by Contemporary Books, Inc.
180 North Michigan Avenue, Chicago, Illinois 60601

To our children, Jim and Kerry

To our mothers,
Maria Photopulos and Kaliope Karabatsos

And to our beloved fathers,
who left us much too soon,
James Photopulos and Mike Karabatsos

Contents

Foreword

The title *Of Tears and Triumphs* expresses in four words the compelling story of a patient with cancer. As one who has long admired Georgia and Bud Photopulos, I am honored to write this foreword. When I met them in January 1972 at an American Cancer Society Education and Crusade conference in New Orleans, Georgia came with a message of valiant struggle, determination, and courage. Then, as now, she said, "When you're fighting cancer you need someone who understands, someone who has not only walked in your shoes, but who is still around leaving footprints." Hers is a gallant story of trust, faith, hope, and love, reaffirming the concept that it is not just that you live but how you live, thus emphasizing the quality of life. This is not merely an account of Georgia and her breast cancer but rather the story of a true partnership between Georgia and Bud, and the effect that her illness had on their lives. It recounts the often searing but more often bonding relationships with family, friends, and physicians. This story is testimony to the triumph of the human spirit in ordeal and reminds us that one must savor even small victories. Her mention of the possibility of recurrence when minor symptoms develop serves as a constant reminder of life's daily challenges and uncertainties.

Major illness constantly tests the strength of a marriage. But it is during moments of adversity that true substance is revealed. Georgia and Bud's resilience compels admiration. Having difficulty adjusting to his mother's illness, Georgia's son told her, "As a mother you have been guilty of only two things—loving too much and trying too hard." This poignant statement reminds us of a mother's attempt to atone for perceived self-inadequacies—whether present or not. The true worth of real friends becomes apparent during times of crisis, as Georgia and Bud found out on numerous occasions.

As a volunteer of the American Cancer Society, Georgia has helped innumerable people. With her background, she has demonstrated an exquisite sensitivity and compassion for others—a true volunteer. She developed a constructive anger that allowed her to be the consummate patient advocate. Appropriately, she emphasizes the need for "fun time" and a sense of humor. Just as strong spiritual faith is needed, so is perseverance with humor.

This book is a true inspiration to us all. But more than anything else, this is a story of hope—a realistic hope, because there is almost always something that can be done to make a patient better. And when we grant patients hope, we grant them one of the greatest of all human joys—the joy of anticipation that perhaps something can be done for them. Georgia and Bud's story is an ideal example of how hope can play such a major role in the fight against cancer. But this is also a story of love, friends, family, and yes, of life itself. Perhaps the French philosopher Teilhard de Chardin expressed it best when he said, "Someday after mastering the winds, the waves, the tides, and gravity, we shall harness for God the energies of love and then for the second time in the history of the world, man shall have discovered fire." It is that love and that fire that this book expresses so well. And Georgia Photopulos is still leaving footprints to help others.

LaSalle D. Leffall, Jr., M.D.
Professor and Chairman
Department of Surgery
Howard University Hospital

Preface

Don't think of this book as an autobiography or as a clinical account of other patients' experiences.

This book is about surviving.

Cancer is one of life's awesome negatives, made more so by attitudes of many who have it and many who treat it. When cancer comes, it disrupts your life, demands huge chunks of time and energy, postpones your plans, reroutes your course, and frequently depletes your savings. It penetrates a family's life fabric as it invades the body, thrusting everyone onto an emotional battleground where tears and heartbreak are confronted daily.

But it can be dealt with. Our experiences and those of thousands of others with whom we've worked show it can be done.

We've written this book because we know what it's like to live with cancer—the feeling, the fear, the anger, the hope, and, sometimes, the lack of hope. In learning how to cope we learned how to give life meaning. In seeking comfort for ourselves we learned how to comfort others.

We found that the human spirit is greater than the forces that attack it and is often the most powerful weapon against them. It can overcome fear, anger, depression. It can give strength, courage and, most of all, hope.

Cancer is a formidable enemy, but it is not invincible. Our refusal to surrender to it enabled us to turn the greatest threat to our lives into our greatest challenge, with rewards far above our expectations.

Our struggle with cancer parallels that of many, many people who must cope with long-term illness. We share our experiences—positive and negative—so that we might provide some measure of support, understanding, and information to those facing similar challenges.

Georgia and Bud Photopulos

Acknowledgments

We wish to acknowledge:

The American Cancer Society for the use of its materials, for believing in our ideas and affording us the opportunity to carry them out.

The National Cancer Institute for their materials, allowing me to add to them, and for inviting me to serve as a consultant.

The Pulitzer Community Newspapers for allowing use of our title, "Of Tears and Triumphs," the name of my columns, and for their permission to reprint material from them.

Our doctors for their professional skills, patience and invaluable advice . . . Ackley, Boxer, Castritsis, Cunningham, Fitzgerald, Galliani, Greenberger, Goldberg, Ilahi, Isaacs, Judd, Karasick, Karkazis, Knaus, Lochman, Nassos, Nathan, O'Connor, Rutgard, and Shavelle.

Our priests and counselors who renewed our strength when we faltered . . . Hondras, Jais, Karloutsos, Kutulas, Lionikis, Murphy, Pekras, Ramseyer, Scoulas, Strouzas, and Thomas.

Janet A. MacKenzie, formerly with the American Cancer Society, a knowledgeable professional with whom we've worked for fifteen years, who assisted us greatly in the preparation of this book.

Nadine Stec, a good friend, who typed the ramblings, notes and fragments that eventually became a manuscript . . . for lost weekends and meeting our deadlines.

Our editor, Susan Buntrock, who listened to our proposal and said, "I'm interested," and provided ongoing support and guidance throughout the project.

And Congdon & Weed/Contemporary Books, Inc., whose faith in us, we trust, has not been misplaced.

For additional acknowledgments, see the Afterword, page 191.

Of Tears and Triumphs

Part One
OUR STORY

1
The Beginning

Bud: We were married by four priests and a bishop in October of 1958. With that kind of ecclesiastical authority around us, it was not difficult to believe that our blessings always would be as great as they were that day, and, in fact, our expectations were high.

Both of us came from immigrant families who worked hard, paid their bills, saved what they could, voted in every election after they gained their citizenship and taught us the "old country" values of faith, loyalty, responsibility.

They never became rich, famous, or powerful, but they were among the most successful people we've ever known. They spoke no English when as children they came from Greece to find that the streets of America were not paved with gold. They found jobs, learned the language, married, survived the Depression, raised their children, and kept their families together.

Our idea of success was to achieve as much as our parents had, and we were looking forward to a life of

3

happiness and fulfillment and, if we were lucky, one
with some financial rewards too.

Each of us had a job that was exciting and challeng-
ing and that had a certain mystique or glamour attached to it. Geo worked for the Federal Bureau of
Investigation in Chicago, assisting agents on security
and criminal investigations and serving as a Greek
interpreter (we can't say more than that). I was a
newswriter and reporter for WBKB (now WLS-TV,
Channel 7), which is the third oldest TV station in the
nation. Occasionally our jobs intertwined when the FBI
would make an arrest and I would cover the story.

Geo: Our honeymoon was the first vacation either of
us had taken; Bud was twenty-five and I was twenty-
four. My family never had a car, so my worldly travel
was limited to a train ride from Council Bluffs, Iowa,
where I was born, to Chicago, Illinois, where I've lived
ever since.

I dreamed of going somewhere romantic, but Bud,
the history buff, had plans of his own. He wanted to go
to Gettysburg, Pennsylvania, and on to Washington,
D.C., if there was no change in his father's condition.
His dad had terminal cancer, so we called home every
day to see if we could continue on our trip.

Gettysburg was a very small town and not as popular
a tourist attraction as it later became. Bud wanted to
retrace the battle, and he was quite disappointed to
learn that I knew little about the Civil War beyond that
it had occurred.

It rained three of the four days we were there. Since
our ten-unit motel didn't have air-conditioning or television (amenities we take for granted today), Bud
thought it was a great opportunity for me to learn about
the war. He bought *A Stillness at Appomattox*, a 484-
page fine-print no-pictures pocket book and insisted
that I read it.

(I got hooked on the war and made Bud promise to
take me back on our first anniversary so that we could
retrace the battle . . . and we did.)

When we went to the Gettysburg Museum, bells clanged and people applauded our arrival. Strange, we thought to ourselves. How did they know we were coming? After the hoopla died down, the director apologized and informed us that we couldn't have the prizes they had just told us were ours. They had made an error and we were not the one-millionth visitors to the museum; we were numbers 999,998 and 999,999. One count away from winning the prize. That's more or less been our situation ever since!

Bud: As soon as we were married, I was assigned to the late shift in the newsroom, working 2:00 P.M. to 11:00 P.M. and not getting home until around midnight. Geo was working 8:00 A.M. to 5:00 P.M. at the bureau. It was as though Cinderella's stepmother had made out our schedules. But closeness was important to us and most of the time Geo would wait around until I was through so we could drive home and be together. About six hours later I'd drive her to work and then go home to try to sleep for a while before heading downtown again.

The powerful forces of youth and love cannot be overestimated!

WBKB at the time had a live show called "Polka-Go-Round" with a polka band, singers, dancers, and an onstage audience that sat at small, candlelit tables to sing along, clap, and stomp their feet to the music. Geo jumped at the chance to become one of the "props." It was a great way for her to wait for me, and whenever I had a break I knew exactly where to find her, getting carried away in Studio B.

When I worked weekends she rocked and rolled with the teenyboppers on Jim Lounsbury's "Record Hop," and on Saturday nights she was a prop on a show called "Marvin's Shock Theater."

My wife, the prop.

Geo: Bud started at WBKB shortly after he was discharged from the army in 1958 and later became the station's first street reporter. In 1965 he moved to the network as a reporter and producer, covering every-

thing from sporting events to space shots, traveling
across the country, sometimes to interesting places
such as New York and Washington, D.C., sometimes
(more often, actually) to less interesting places such as
Iola, Kansas (population: 7,000).

Despite his distaste for flying, he loved the work, and
we enjoyed it too. Many times I got the children ready,
packed their diapers and formulas on an hour's notice,
and we went with him, paying our own way, of course.
That gave us a sense of participation in his work and
helped maintain the closeness that was so important to
us.

Once Bud was covering a Lincoln Day observance in
Springfield, Illinois, where Senate minority leader Ev-
erett Dirksen was the principal speaker.

At the senator's news conference afterward I asked
Bud why Dirksen didn't comb his long, silvery hair,
which, because of its eternal messiness, had become a
trademark for him, along with his mellifluous voice and
oratorical style of speaking.

The senator overheard me, and as Bud tried to find a
hole to fall into, he smiled and said, "But I do, my dear,
I do." News conferences were off limits to me after that.

Bud: Eventually I was assigned to a newly created
extra-late shift, 5:00 P.M. to 1:00 A.M. By this time Geo
had resigned from the bureau. We didn't enjoy being
apart every evening, but professionally it was one of the
best things that ever happened to me. Our anchorman
at the time was Alex Dreier, "The Man on the Go," and I
was assigned to help his writer-producer, Don Bresna-
han, prepare the late-night newscast. I mention their
names because they and our enormously popular news-
caster, Paul Harvey, taught me more about our profession of reporting news and producing newscasts than
everyone else in the last thirty years.

Had I not been assigned to that late shift, I might not
have had the opportunity to learn from them.

Geo: It was suggested to Bud that he might want to
shorten his name for professional purposes, and I

thought of a great one. Chet Huntley and David Brinkley were the hottest thing in the news business, and I thought that since Bud was part of Alex's team, they could be known as Washer (Bud) and Dreier. Everyone laughed—but Bud kept his last name.

Bud: My father died less than three months after our marriage, thrusting me into a new role as head of the family. That meant helping to provide for my mother, grandmother, and teenaged sister, all of whom urged us to move in with them to cut down on expenses. We resisted that.

The construction boom had not yet begun, and finding a place to live, especially one we could afford, had been difficult. We were fortunate to find a small third-floor apartment on a main thoroughfare. We found out why the first night we tried to sleep there. Just across the street was a post office. We knew that, but we didn't know they loaded their trucks all night long. The banging, pounding, and clanging, as the mailbags were thrown onto the metal trucks, drove us crazy. It was a nightly ritual that robbed us of our sleep and helped create the insomnia that has plagued us both ever since.

But Geo and I steadfastly refused to give up our small place to move in with my family even though it would have been cheaper . . . and quieter. We were going to do everything possible to preserve our closeness and privacy.

Geo: There were five more deaths in our immediate family within a two-year period, so there wasn't too much joy around us. More and more, we drew our strength from each other.

We adopted Jimmy in November of 1962, when he was a month old. He was a bright, precocious child and brought the entire family much happiness. Alex Dreier surprised us by sending a camera crew to the adoption agency as Bud and I officially welcomed Baby Photopulos to our family. It was the day before Thanksgiving, and it made our holiday a very special one.

After my dad died in the spring of 1964, we decided

to buy a house so that we'd have room for the second child we hoped to adopt and, if necessary, for our mothers now that both were widowed.

Bud: Shortly after that I moved over to ABC's Midwest Bureau in Chicago and was earning enough to enable us to buy a bilevel house in the city. We adopted our daughter, Kerry, in April of 1966 and were beginning to look like a typical midwestern family—a house, two cars, two children. Except for my erratic hours, our life was beginning to take on a semblance of normalcy . . . and we planned to live happily ever after.

It didn't quite work out that way. It wasn't long before our expectations of living the "American Dream" were shattered.

Geo: In 1965 I discovered that I was bleeding from the nipple of my right breast. My doctor diagnosed it as fibrocystic disease and removed a large section of diseased tissue.

But the bleeding continued, then appeared in the other breast, and I had four operations in three months. When the time came for the second one, we decided to consult other doctors. Their recommendations ranged from doing nothing to removing both breasts immediately.

This last suggestion was one that neither Bud nor I was prepared to accept. Looking back, though, it probably was the best because, eventually, that's exactly what happened. But at the time we decided to undergo each operation as it was deemed necessary.

My health had to be watched carefully when I was growing up. I contracted polio at eleven and have a crooked pelvis and curvature of the spine as battle scars. I've always had allergies and asthma and had undergone surgery several times before, so when the recurrent surgeries for fibrocystic disease came along, I was not particularly distressed.

These problems came on the heels of a long series of treatments to correct a hormone imbalance. Bud and I longed to have children, so I went through a sterility work-up. After two miscarriages, I was given weekly injections of estrogen. When nothing seemed to work, I was given birth control pills, not to prevent pregnancy but to encourage it.

For a while things went relatively well. Then in early September of 1968 both children were hospitalized, Kerry with convulsions resulting from an extremely high fever, Jimmy with salmonella poisoning.

On the day Jimmy came home, September 21, I conducted a self-examination of my breasts, as I had been doing regularly.

I froze! My fingers had found two small, hard lumps, one in my right underarm, the other in the breast itself.

Oddly enough, Bud had just covered a seminar on cancer for ABC and had brought home a number of pamphlets. One of them was on breast cancer. I read it over and over again. Then, my fingers trembling from fear, I repeated the exam. The lumps were there, all right.

Another wave of fear surged through me. I thought of all our friends and close relatives we had lost to cancer. Try as I would, I could not think of anyone I knew who had survived. Oh, some names came to mind—John Wayne, Arthur Godfrey, and Virginia Graham—but most celebrities can afford the best medical care. I couldn't think of anyone with limited resources who was living a full and productive life.

Not wanting to alarm Bud yet, I called my gynecologist, and he saw me immediately. His feeling was that the lumps indeed were different from the earlier fibrocystic disease, but he told me to wait the three weeks until my next menstrual period to see if they might disappear.

Convinced that I could expect more surgery, I left his office desperately needing someone to talk to. I called several friends and expressed my fears to them, but they all said: "Don't worry, I'm sure it won't be anything serious. Anyway, I'm busy now." I was not only terribly depressed and frightened but deeply hurt as well.

Then I remembered a place where I would be welcomed, a place where I could leave my problems and find peace of mind. I drove directly to church. Bud and I are Greek Orthodox. My family, my life, my church— I can't separate them.

I knelt in the serene setting for more than an hour, praying, crying, talking aloud. I asked God to lead me and give me strength. I had never been a bitter person, and I made a kind of "arrangement" with God.

I would, of course, accept whatever lay ahead— surgery, pain, whatever His plan for me entailed. I promised that if I lived I would continue to be a loving wife and a devoted mother, and that I would become a source of inspiration to sick and sorrowing people.

Finally I went home, my mind clear, ready to tell Bud and to help him adjust to the news.

After he had helped me put the children to bed that night, Bud sensed my anxiety and asked what was wrong. I told him. He seemed stunned, and his eyes filled with tears.

Then I remembered a beautiful thought Bud had written in a Bible he had given me one Christmas Eve, the night before he asked me to marry him: "Perfect love casteth out fear."

Suddenly I was babbling on about how lucky we were, how I could endure whatever it was, how we would never leave one another.

Bud nodded, and in a voice filled with emotion he told me that losing a breast would not change the girl he had married. It would not, he said, alter my compassion, intelligence or personality. His understanding gave me an immediate feeling of relief and confidence.

In our marriage, sometimes I had been the strong one, sometimes Bud. But that night, as we held and comforted each other, we assured ourselves that we would fight this thing together. We were approaching ten years of marriage, and we had encountered enough adversity to topple even the most strong-willed of people—major illness, deaths of parents and relatives, financial worries, miscarriages—but, thank God, no marital problems.

I reminded myself that night of how much I had to be grateful for. I had a marvelous husband, and together we had a unique relationship. He was intelligent, sincere, strong, reflective, as his baptismal name of Socrates implied. I was talkative and outgoing, with a quick sense of humor that had helped to pull us through many adversities.

Now not only my own life was being threatened at thirty-four years of age; so was our lifestyle. I resolved not to let it happen.

In the weeks that followed, whomever I tried to talk to about my fear gave me the same reply: "Don't worry, relax. I'm sure it's nothing serious." That's when I first realized that cancer creates such anxiety that no one wants to talk about it.

The three weeks dragged by, filled with tension. The lumps were still there. The recommendation was immediate surgery.

Bud: As we waited out the three weeks, I emulated the well-known practice of my favorite baseball team, the Chicago Cubs, who would go into a funk sometime around June and stay that way until September. My own June swoon was a refusal, at first, to face the situation. I kept hoping the lumps would go away, that somehow they would disappear and the threat they carried would cease to exist.

Of course, I knew that this was only wishful thinking, but that's about all I was capable of then. I think psychiatrists call this denial, and I was a textbook case.

But you can deny only so long, and when I finally realized the lumps were not going to go away by themselves, I broke out of my stupor and began a frantic search for whatever information there was on the subject, looking primarily, I admit, for something positive, something that would say everything was going to be all right.

The most hopeful information I could find was that if breast cancer was detected in its earliest stages and was treated promptly and properly, there was some hope for survival.

I hit the libraries; I talked to doctors; I read the literature of the American Cancer Society. Nowhere did I find anything encouraging.

In fact, there was darn little for the layman. (This was 1968, remember.) I found not a word about radiation, not a word about chemotherapy, not a word about survivors. After all my research, I knew little more than I had before.

I was angry and frustrated because I desperately needed something to pin my hopes on, some evidence that the miracles of science we all had been hearing about could be used to cure my wife's illness.

Geo: Remembering the advice I had received two years earlier, I asked that both breasts be removed, even if the lumps turned out to be benign. The answer was no. A radical mastectomy would be performed on the right side *only* if the lumps were malignant.

On October 8, 1968, I entered the hospital for surgery the following day. All the rooms were filled, and I was told I'd have to spend the night in a small conference room equipped with a spare bed.

That disappointed me. I'm a perfectionist—hard-driving, compulsive, organized. I take pride in the research and organizational abilities I learned at the FBI. I live by a daily work list attached to a large calendar, and I hadn't overlooked anything in preparing for a hospital stay of undetermined days.

The children had been provided for. I had made lists for Bud, left him notes, and even had Halloween costumes ready for the children in case I wouldn't be home by then.

I had tried to explain to the children about my surgery and my absence from home by telling them that if they needed me I was just a phone call away. So when I was told I'd be in a room without a phone, I was dismayed.

There was one thing more. I'm sure other women faced with this situation understand my feelings and what motivated me to do it.

I bought a beautiful anniversary card and wrote Bud a farewell love letter telling him how much he meant to me and that if I didn't survive, I wanted him to remarry. But, being honest, I said I didn't want anyone better to replace me. I wanted someone who would clean and cook, be nice and kind and not terribly attractive.

I placed the card and letter in my drawer, along with instructions that they should be opened October 19, 1968—our tenth wedding anniversary—if . . .

Bud drove me to the hospital, stopping first at church to say a prayer and then at the home of Kerry's godparents, Fran and Nick Mechales, who were having a birthday party for their little daughter, Stacey. We left the children playing happily there.

They weren't kidding when they said there was no room at the hospital. I found myself in a combination conference room and supply room, where constant activity made it impossible for Bud and me to be alone. At 9:15 P.M. Bud left, exhausted and worried.

It was then that I got out the medical encyclopedia and brochures I had sneaked in and devoured them like a teenager with a dirty book. I studied a diagram of a radical mastectomy and read every word carefully so that I would not be surprised if I returned from surgery minus one breast.

I read that if cancer was caught when it was still confined to the milk duct of the breast, the chances of surviving for five years were pretty high, more than 90 percent, but they dropped to only 50 percent if it had spread to the lymph nodes underneath the arms. I also read that premenopausal women with breast cancer did not survive as long as those who had passed menopause.

To me that meant the younger you are the worse it is, a horrible thought to contemplate while awaiting surgery.

A radical mastectomy was the treatment of choice for breast cancer in 1968. Since then, lumpectomies, modified mastectomies, and simple mastectomies have become more common for very early cancer detected by low-dose mammography.

As they wheeled me away the next morning, Bud walked alongside me, holding my hand. The big doors marked "Surgery" swung open. Bud kissed me good-bye and managed a thin smile.

Bud: Although the next five hours are not in Geo's memory bank, they are very much in mine. My mother, my uncle, several close friends, and our priest had offered to wait out the surgery with me, but I asked them not to come.

I wanted to be alone, to wait it out by myself, so that I wouldn't have to pretend I was brave if the news was bad. I tried to read a book I had brought along, but even though it was on my favorite subject, history, I couldn't get into it. I looked through several magazines. Later, I couldn't remember what they were.

I sat a little. I paced a little. I prayed a lot.

In what I thought was an amazingly short period of time the doctors came out to talk to me, and I thought they had good news, but then I realized they weren't smiling. They told me they'd removed three lumps and made frozen sections. The first two were benign, the last malignant. "We'll have to remove the breast," one said. "Is that all right with you?"

Heck no, it wasn't all right. It wasn't what I wanted to hear. It was, however, what I had feared, and I nodded my approval. They returned to the operating room, and I sat down to wait some more.

Geo: When they returned me to my room, Bud was

there, waiting. I was not so groggy that I failed to see him. And I wanted to be alert for another reason. We never had kept any secrets from each other, and we wouldn't now.

"Was it malignant?" I asked.

Bud nodded sadly and said, "Yes."

I asked if it had spread to the lymph nodes.

Again he nodded yes.

Bud: I spent as much time as I could with Geo in the recovery room, stretching the five-minute-per-hour limit until the nurses ran me out of the room. I would hang around the hospital until the next visiting period rolled around, sometimes going to the coffee shop, sometimes sitting in the lobby, sometimes wandering the halls in the aimless manner of a man who had nowhere to go but who had all the time in the world to get there.

One day I ran into someone I knew, someone with whom I had worked in the period between my graduation from college and my induction into the army. Both of us had been caught in a Selective Service squeeze play. With universal military service the law of the land during the Korean Conflict, employers were unwilling to hire anyone who had not completed his tour of duty, and we found ourselves working at a downtown department store, he as a necktie salesman, I as a floor manager, until the army decided it had room for us.

I hadn't seen him for more than a dozen years, but there he was, walking the hospital halls, just as I was. After shaking hands and saying hello, we asked each other what we were doing there. I told him why I was there, and I expected his answer would be similar to mine—that someone in his family was ill.

"Oh, no," he said. "I'm a doctor."

It didn't exactly fill me with confidence to know that my friend, the necktie salesman, was now a doctor at the hospital where my wife was being treated for cancer.

I didn't mean to question my friend's competence as a

doctor, but the difference in our situations couldn't have struck me at a worse time. He had been turned down by the army, gone to medical school, and was now a practicing physician, on the way, I guessed, to the upper tax brackets.

I, on the other hand, had served two years in the army, had passed up graduate school because of my father's terminal illness, and now was trying to cope with the news that my wife had come down with the same disease that had claimed my father's life.

I was anything but brave at that time, but I still was hopeful because I didn't fully understand the nature of the disease and because I was engaging in some wishful thinking that the surgery, like a mother's kiss, had made Geo's illness go away.

Our decision not to permit cancer to overrun our lives was made early and possibly without conscious effort. Geo was still in the hospital when the Kidney Foundation of Illinois gave me an award for a story I had done on home kidney dialysis. They called the office to notify me and were given the number of Geo's hospital room. When she heard who it was on the phone, she kiddingly asked if I had donated one of her kidneys now that she had lost a breast. I'm not sure that the person on the other end knew he was calling a hospital, but he assured Geo that he not only didn't want her kidneys but wanted to invite us to the awards presentation at the Palmer House hotel.

I thanked them for selecting me for the honor and explained that I wouldn't be able to attend the dinner because of Geo's surgery. But she told her doctor about that call and begged him to let her go. He said there was no reason she couldn't if she followed all of his instructions. He said he would give her a six-hour pass, so long as she was back at the hospital by 11:00 P.M., when the nursing shift changed.

The day of the dinner was an exciting one for Geo as she prepared for the trip downtown. With friends, relatives, and nurses all pitching in, we got her dressed, made up, and ready to go. This was only five days after her surgery, so we tied her hemo-vac to a wheel chair, covered it with the folds of her dress, sat her down, and off we went to the party.

We had a beautiful evening together, and when it was over I drove her back to the hospital, happy to have had a brief time with her. We managed to return in time for Geo's medication.

Geo: I felt like Cinderella, all dressed up and waiting for my prince. On the way downtown I begged Bud to stop by the house so I could see the children. They were only two and five years old and weren't allowed up in my hospital room. They were so excited—they ran out to the car, and we hugged and cried. We had to hurry so that Bud could be at the dinner on time, and as we pulled away I remember praying quietly, "Please God, please let me live to see them grow."

Bud: It wasn't until Geo was undergoing radiation therapy that I began to get an idea of the long and torturous path we had ahead of us. I would wait in the radiation lounge while she underwent some of her treatments of deep x-ray and cobalt therapy. The lounge was anything but. It reminded me of pictures I had seen of the London subways during World War II, where people huddled together, waiting out the German air raids, fear, helplessness, and desperation etched on their faces.

Every day I would wait, watching the bleak expressions of the other people in the lounge, knowing my own was just as bleak.

I thumbed through some of the magazines I found there but was unable to concentrate long enough to read any of them until I came across an article in the *Reader's Digest*, one of those first-person accounts written, of course, by a *Digest* writer, in this case a man who later did a story about Georgia, Walter Ross.

It was a touching, tear-jerking story of a man whose

wife had had breast cancer. It told of her repeated
hospitalizations, surgeries, and treatment. It was then
that I began to understand that cancer was not something confined to a single episode, cured by a single
operation. The doctors had not prepared me for that.

The story did not have a happy ending. The wife died,
and I was devastated. It had blown away my fantasy
that everything was going to be all right as soon as
Geo's radiation was finished.

The man in the story was portrayed as facing his
wife's death with strength and courage, two qualities of
which I was in short supply. When I put down the
magazine I was crying, trembling and scared to death,
and perhaps, worst of all, I was unable to offer comfort
or support to Geo as she left the clinic that day, fighting
off the pain, nausea, and weakness caused by the accumulated treatments.

Geo: That was only the beginning of many difficult
years of pain, surgery, and long absences from home.
But they were also years of hope, for I refused to give in
to despair, steeling myself in faith that gave me courage and dissipated my pain.

Following my partial recovery from surgery, I was
sent as an outpatient to a radiation clinic. I received a
combination of 120 treatments of deep x-ray and cobalt
therapy. They made me nauseated. As the number of
treatments increased, I could barely swallow. The pain
and discomfort grew. My skin reddened, both on the
chest and on the back. The combined treatments
burned and penetrated deeply.

It was torture to lie beneath the giant cobalt machine,
my arm strapped above my head, the pain from the
incision searing through me. Not only the breast had
been removed but the underlying chest muscles as well,
along with the lymph glands that drain it. That's what
they mean by a radical mastectomy—it's extreme. Because of the preceding surgeries and resultant scar
tissue, so much skin had had to be cut away that the

skin from my back had to be pulled very taut to close the incision.

My skin fit so tightly I could barely breathe. Standing up straight was impossible. My pronounced curvature of the right shoulder, resulting from my bout with polio, was greatly aggravated. I was in constant pain.

Despite all of this, I had to lie motionless beneath the cobalt machine. I prayed as I lay there and asked the person who had driven me for treatment to pray for me. I visited the hospital chapel before every treatment and again afterward to say "Thanks, God, for getting me through another day." It would have been easy to give up. But life is worth fighting for, and I fought as hard as I could.

Finally the treatments were completed. But the discomfort, the burns, the scars, and the pain remained for some time.

I went in for regular examinations in the months that followed, and I seemed to be healing normally. Friends and strangers alike responded with kindness, offering help with the children and rides to the doctor. Some worried openly about me, and a few even offered miracle cures, ranging from Indian herb tea to Krebiozen, a substance derived from the blood of certain horses.

Bud: Before Krebiozen was discredited in the early sixties it had gained some credence because its chief exponent was a distinguished and respected doctor from the University of Illinois, Andrew C. Ivy, who staked his reputation and career on it. I remember it particularly because its developers were indicted for fraud and conspiracy and I covered part of the trial.

I was moved by the scores of people who demonstrated at the courthouse, saying Krebiozen cured them of cancer. This was several years before Geo became ill. Although the trial resulted in no convictions, Krebiozen was discredited and soon forgotten. Still, I'll never forget those people who demonstrated. I can't explain why they thought they'd been cured, but I do know that

many patients when desperate, try anything, are willing to believe in anything that promises a cure, and
often find it difficult to see things for what they really
are.

Geo: These things disturbed us. We knew that there
was no known cure, except for early detection, if that
can be considered a cure. Mine had been caught early,
but how could we be sure it was early enough? We
decided to go to the Mayo Clinic at Rochester, Minne-
sota, now known as the Mayo Medical Center, for a
thorough checkup. It was as though Providence had
guided us.

Bud: The Mayo Clinic is a fascinating place, a sprawl-
ing complex of diagnostic machinery and a great repos-
itory of medical knowledge, wisdom, and skill. There
are also two huge hospitals, St. Mary's and Methodist,
where all of that is put to work to save lives.

It probably saved Geo's life. She underwent her second mastectomy there, even though all of the tests run
on her were negative, thanks to the wisdom of Dr.
Edward Judd, an outstanding surgeon and a direct
descendant of the Mayo brothers. He told us the breast
had at least a 20 percent chance of becoming cancerous
and recommended its removal. I'll never forget Geo's
reaction. She didn't hesitate a moment. "How about
tomorrow?" she said.

Less than twenty-four hours later she was in surgery
again at St. Mary's Hospital, and when the pathology
report came back it showed that a small tumor was,
indeed, in the breast. I don't want to think about what
might have happened had the tumor not been detected
until it had grown and perhaps spread. I know that,
with the emphasis today on lumpectomy and other
procedures, some surgeons and laymen will think the
procedure performed on Geo was radical and perhaps
unnecessarily deforming. But we have no second
guesses, no misgivings, and are, in fact, thankful it was
done.

St. Mary's was a great hospital, but not a fun place to hang around in. It was, first of all, old. Geo's room was dreary. It needed a paint job. The plumbing was antiquated. There was no TV set. There was nothing to take your mind off your pain.

For the first few days after her surgery, Geo slept most of the time, the painkillers making her drowsy, and I sat next to her all day long, wishing there were tiles on the ceiling so I could count them.

One day I discovered a wonderful way to pass the time and take my thoughts off her illness. I bought a book of crossword puzzles and started to fill in the blanks. I had never done them before—after all, they weren't nearly as much fun as playing baseball—but I soon became addicted to the little squares. They occupied my mind and hands for hours, making me think a little but not insisting that I retain anything, something like a coloring book for grown-ups, and that's about all I could handle.

Geo: When I was well enough to get out of bed, Bud helped me into a wheelchair, and together we made the long trip down the elevator and through the endless maze of corridors of St. Mary's Hospital to the chapel. The intravenous paraphernalia clattered behind us, along with the old-fashioned breast drainage pump and the catheter bag, as we rattled our way to give thanks that we had discovered this new malignancy before it had had time to grow.

Bud: On July 20, 1969, Neil Armstrong became the first man to walk on the moon. This dramatic fulfillment of the manned space program's mission dominated the newspapers, the airwaves, and the conversation everywhere you went.

But in July of 1969 Georgia and I had been getting ready for our trip to Mayo and quite frankly, we couldn't have cared less. Our minds were not on the moon or what Armstrong's landing on it meant, but on what our trip to Mayo would mean to us. Many people

remember where they were and what they were doing
when important events took place—Pearl Harbor, V-J
Day, President Kennedy's assassination—and many
people, I'm sure, remember the day Neil Armstrong
took that "giant step for mankind," but I don't. I read
about it, I heard about it, but I don't remember it, and
the only reason I know it happened around the time we
were at Mayo is that I had to cover a parade in Armstrong's honor soon after we returned.

Geo: We spent two weeks in Rochester and went home
confident the worst was over. But in another two weeks
a lump appeared on the right side of my throat. It was
removed and found to be benign.

A few weeks after that still another appeared, this
one on the chest wall on the right side. It was malignant.

We were terrified once more, and Bud telephoned Dr.
Judd to tell him what had happened and to ask if we
should return to Rochester. He'd be happy to treat me,
he said, but he felt I was in able hands here at home if
we chose not to make the trip.

We were sure of that also, and since I was weak and
we were short of money, we decided to stay home.

My doctors decided then that the next step should be
the removal of my ovaries to reduce the supply of estrogen, which they thought might be contributing to the
formation of the lesions. The oophorectomy took place
in October of 1969.

Bud: So, in less than three months, Geo had undergone four more surgeries and was exhausted. I was too.
She was unable to go up and down the stairs in our
home. She was very weak and needed someone with her
constantly. I had used up all of my vacation and a leave
of absence as well and could not take any more time.

Georgia's mother came in from Tulsa to be with her,
and her sister, Chrissy, and Chrissy's husband, Phil,
offered to look after the children at their home in Florida. I was unwilling to accept their offer at first because

I didn't want the children to be separated from us, but I soon decided they would be better off there, playing and going to school with their cousins, John and Karen, than they would be staying in the tense and depressing atmosphere of our house. Money was so tight, though, what with our medical bills and my being away from work, that we couldn't afford the airfare.

While I was considering ways to raise the money, our good friends Sam and Georgia Booras presented us with airline tickets and told me to get moving. I was overwhelmed by their generosity and concern, put aside my pride, and took Jim and Kerry to Tampa.

By Christmas Geo had recovered enough so that we could fly to Florida to pick them up and bring them home again. We found Jimmy to be the same; in fact, he enjoyed his visit. But Kerry, who had always been a picky eater, began overeating, gained ten pounds in eight weeks, and looked like a little chipmunk. Jimmy was six and was in the first grade, and Kerry, who was only three, attended nursery school there. We were afraid she wouldn't recognize us, but the children hugged us tightly, and the four of us had a tearful reunion kneeling on the floor of Chrissy's living room at two o'clock in the morning.

We spent two weeks with Chrissy's family, away from the turmoil of the preceding months, taking advantage of our first opportunity to rest and defuse the highly charged atmosphere we were living in.

Our stay there was helpful in another, unexpected way. We were introduced to an oncologist—a specialist in tumors. We hadn't known such a specialist existed, but we made it our first order of business when we returned home to find one.

There weren't many, fewer than a hundred throughout the nation. Oncology was a new specialty at the time and oncologists weren't listed as such in the phone book. We called the American Cancer Society and the American Medical Association, where Geo had worked before

going to the FBI, for guidance. We found Dr. Myles
Cunningham and put ourselves in his care.

It was one of the best things we ever did! He told Geo
she would have to be under continual medical surveil-
lance for the rest of her life with regular exams and
tests that, although inconvenient, were essential to
monitoring her condition and discovering anything that
might develop at an early stage.

Far from considering it an inconvenience, we were
happy he was taking charge and calling the shots. We
felt we were in good hands, and our confidence was
restored.

In April 1970, when Geo experienced vaginal bleeding, unusual since she had no ovaries, Dr. Cunningham
sent her to a gynecologist who specialized in treating
cancer patients. His test in May of 1970 indicated the
bleeding was being caused by fibroid tumors in the
uterus, and he recommended an immediate hysterectomy.

At the same time, though, Geo discovered a hard and
painful lump near the incision on the left side of her
chest wall and that took precedence. It was removed
and, to our great relief, it turned out to be scar tissue
only.

A few days later Geo underwent a complete hysterectomy, major surgery under the most favorable circumstances. Coming as it did after the long series of operations she had undergone during a period of just a few
months, the hysterectomy left Geo weaker than she had
ever been. We were happy that no malignancy was
found, but we were physically worn out and emotionally
exhausted. Geo spent most of the summer in a wheelchair and I spent much of it worrying about her.

By fall she had recovered. The surgery was successful. The bleeding had stopped.

2
When the Crisis Is Over
. . . or Seems to Be

Bud: After her hysterectomy, Geo's situation shifted from a series of crises to a chronic condition and was a matter of dealing not so much with recurrences as with the fear of recurrences. It was impossible not to think of any physical problem, no matter how slight, as evidence of a new cancer. Once Geo scratched the inside of her ear without realizing it; when we saw it bleeding, we were so terrified we got our friend and neighbor, Dr. Mike Govostis, out of bed to look at it right away. Every headache, every stomachache, every cut had sinister implications, and it was a very long time before we learned to identify them for what they were.

I'd read somewhere that medical students recognize in themselves the symptoms of whatever disease they happen to be studying. Now I understand why.

Geo saw her doctors—and by then we had built up quite a collection—regularly undergoing exams, probings, blood tests, x-rays, hoping to stay on top of her condition or, better yet, to keep one step ahead. It was a

25

painful, energy-sapping, time-consuming and expensive process, but one that had to be pursued.

Senator Barry Goldwater once said that eternal vigilance is the price of liberty. He might have added of life itself. He might have said it takes a lot of money, too.

That's something a lot of people don't understand, especially if they haven't been ill or responsible for someone's long-term medical care. Insurance doesn't cover everything; there were a lot of extra expenses related to medical care that most people wouldn't think about. Parking fees, for example, or cab fares, baby-sitters, meals eaten outside the home, telephone calls from a hospital room or pay booth, and hotel rooms if treatment is sought away from home.

Insurance pays for none of these. Nor does it pay for tipping someone to do something for you so you can zip over to the hospital or provide the extra money you might pay to buy a new pair of shoes for one of the kids because you don't have the time or energy to shop around for the best price.

These expenses, like the federal deficit, have a way of adding up, and you may not realize it until you try to balance your checkbook at the end of the month.

We've heard many patients recite this tale of the declining bank account, complaining not that they have to spend the money but that their friends or relatives don't seem to understand they don't have much left over for other things.

People constantly asked us, "How come you can't go out to dinner with us?" "Why don't you go to concerts or the opera anymore?" "What do you expect when you buy cheap or used cars? You should buy more expensive ones so that they don't break down all the time." "Why don't you send your children away to summer camp?" "Why don't you have household help?"

Few cancer patients get totally out from under the avalanche of their medically related bills. They do get some financial relief, however, as their physical condition improves. We found that a period of relatively good health means less money is allocated to hospital and doctor bills and more is available for other things, enabling families to resume activities that had been sacrificed.

We made a point of going away for a few days or a week over Labor Day, usually to a vacation lodge in Wisconsin where the kids had plenty to keep them occupied and we could relax. The timing was important. It was a pleasant way to end the summer, and the kids could go back to school with happy memories. Once, after Geo's sister and her family had moved to California, we took a train trip to Los Angeles, something I'd always wanted to do when I was a boy, and the three kids in the family—Jim, Kerry, and I—had a great time. The ride was a little too bumpy for Geo, though, so we flew back.

As Geo got better, we were able to do things with our friends again. Our cancer-related activities had introduced us to many new ones; she had resumed driving, which gave her independence; my career seemed to be on an upswing; and, even though we could not keep from worrying about her health, we were happy.

Our relative calm was shattered, however, when we received a kidnap threat on Jimmy, then in the fifth grade.

We notified the police, of course, and they kept an eye on both children, following them to and from school. To protect them from being snatched from the playground, the officers kept them inside during recess and made sure they didn't play after school. Every day Jim was given a set of instructions. Every day for almost three months, he and Kerry had to stay indoors or be accompanied by an adult wherever they went.

Kerry didn't seem to mind, content to read or play with her dolls. Jimmy, though, bursting with energy and eager to play with the other boys, resented the confinement. Other parents, fearing their own children might be kidnapped, were reluctant to let them come to our house to play.

Most of our friends were certain the threat had come because we had made a number of television appearances for the American Cancer Society and had, therefore, achieved a certain celebrity. But it hadn't. While the police never arrested anyone, their investigation determined that threats also had been directed at three other adolescent boys in the school who had been adopted and who lived in the immediate area.

The threat was cruel, despicable, heartless. It added to the considerable degree of tension that already existed in our house, and it drove away some of our friends who, whether fearing for their children's safety, or that our run of misfortune might be contagious, simply never have been heard from since.

Our next crisis occurred in the spring of 1977. We were going along pretty well and were even managing to rebuild our bank account when I found myself on strike. I belong to two unions, one of which permits me to write and produce (NABET), the other to appear on the air (AFTRA). Not everyone belongs to two unions, but many people do, and in a previous year when both unions struck at the same time, those of us who do found ourselves sitting on a barbed-wire fence. The company would send telegrams to AFTRA members telling us we were under contract and had to report to work or be terminated. That would be followed by another telegram from AFTRA ordering us not to go to work or face disciplinary action.

One day, when the doorbell rang at 6:00 A.M., I went to the door expecting another offer I couldn't refuse. Instead, it was a special-delivery letter from an old army buddy who said he, his wife, and his four kids were on their way to spend ten days with us and were, in fact, arriving that very same day. I was in no mood to receive them, especially since we had seen them during a vacation not too long before, had been invited to their home for dinner, and when we got there were offered neither dinner nor even a glass of water.

I was furious. I began thinking up ways to keep them out. I considered putting up a quarantine sign on the door. I considered moving in with my mother. I considered shooting him. Then I realized that Geo was taking the news much too calmly, and eventually she admitted she had arranged for her sister to send the letter from another state as a joke to cheer me up. I didn't think it was funny then, not since I was on strike and had no income, but today I can laugh at it.

Sort of.

When the second NABET strike dragged into its tenth week or so (it lasted twenty), I felt I had to find some kind of work to keep our bank account from being depleted again. I wound up delivering telephone books and recruited the entire family to help me. Geo was so eager she asked the distributor to let us have the entire north side of Chicago—more than a million five-pound phone books that had to be run up and down stairs and dropped at every subscriber's door. Fortunately, the distributor was wiser than we were and gave us a much smaller area. We filled both our cars with phone books and, bumpers dragging, started out to deliver them in one-hundred-degree heat. That career lasted about two days. We couldn't continue. We had delivered thousands of books and had earned the grand sum of $88.64.

That episode was just a measure of my desperation, which prevented me from thinking clearly. Later I was able to place a few articles I had written (one in *Newsweek*), which earned me considerably more than the going rate for delivering a million phone books. The phone book experience, however, was another lesson in how much we need the support of our families. For years I had supported mine. Now they had supported me, even in a misguided effort.

Some say our trials bring us closer together. They miss the point. It's our closeness that brings us through trials together.

Things returned to normal rather quickly after the strike, and Geo's overall health remained good, but her energy was being sapped by the house we lived in. It had three levels: the bedrooms and a bathroom on the upper level; the dining room, living room, and kitchen on the main level; and the den, laundry area, and another bathroom on the bottom level. Going up and down the stairs was becoming increasingly difficult and painful for Geo since she suffered from arthritis as a side effect of her illness.

Doctors had ordered her not to go up and down stairs, but there was no way to avoid them in our house unless she stayed in the bedroom all day. Making one trip down to the kitchen and one trip up to the bedroom wouldn't have been so bad except for the fact that she would have had to go up or down to get to the bathroom and then down or up to get back to the kitchen. Is it possible that the people who design and build homes never get sick? Or don't they ever have to go to the bathroom?

We installed one of those expensive devices that let you ride up and down, but because of the design of our stairways, it worked on only one set of stairs. It didn't help much.

Parking also was a problem. Since many families have two or more cars these days, there seldom was a parking space near our house, and Geo often had to park several blocks away. We built a parking slab in the backyard, but that was of little use in the wintertime when the alley was filled with snow and wasn't plowed.

We decided the only option was to sell the house. We moved into a one-level condominium with a garage three days before the presidential election of 1980. We had planned to move in May of that year, but couldn't because of construction delays.

Iran was still holding its American hostages, but there were recurring reports that they soon would be released. Though the rumors were false (the hostages weren't set free until President Reagan's Inauguration Day in January 1981), all news organizations were kept busy checking them out while at the same time covering the final days of the campaign.

I was able to take only one day off, but again close friends came to our rescue. They helped us pack, unpack, and put things into some type of order after the movers left.

We were the first family to move into our building of seventy units. The lobby, corridors, and garage were unfinished. Workmen swarmed through the building. Our telephone wasn't installed for another three weeks. But we'd had to vacate our house, so we pressured the builder to complete our first-floor apartment in time for our move.

I didn't like the circumstances but had little choice. Fortunately, the children were old enough to help Geo and fend for themselves.

Our 25th anniversary in 1983 was a time of genuine celebration.

We had reached a plateau; for the first time in our married life things seemed to be under control. Jim had finished school and was working; Kerry was a senior in high school. Most important of all, Geo had had only a few skirmishes with her health, the worst of which was a severe reaction to an allergy shot. The resulting anaphylactic shock sent her to the hospital once again. She was in danger of dying, but quick intervention by her allergist, Bob Boxer, saved her life.

It was a freak thing and, unlike her previous medical problems, something we could stop worrying about as soon as it was over.

Her painful arthritic condition had greatly improved, she had resumed driving, and all in all, she felt relatively well.

We had another reason to celebrate: Geo's original prognosis had made the probability of reaching our 25th anniversary highly unlikely, but we had made it.

We had beaten the odds!

We wanted everyone who had been a part of our survival to be part of our celebration, so we invited them to a party in the hall of Saint Andrew's Greek Orthodox Church, where my faith in God had taken root and where we both had received sustenance and support in our fight against cancer. We invited friends of our parents, friends of Kerry's, and friends of Jim's. Jim had just turned twenty-one, and we made it his party as well. In all, there were almost six hundred people—our doctors, our priests, our cancer "buddies."

Our bishop brought along twenty-five members of a visiting youth group to show them, as he said, what a successful marriage really was. We didn't know if we should be flattered or upset, but in a crowd of six hundred, what difference did another twenty-five make?

I gave a short speech, saying there had been a strong chance that both of us would not be around to see that night but that through the grace of God and with the help of some wonderful doctors we were. I wanted to say a lot more, but my eyes filled with tears and I could not go on.

The party did, though, and we enjoyed a wonderful evening, forgetting for a few hours the illness and other problems that had come before. Life had to go on, too. We could not change the events of the past, but we were not going to be held prisoner by them, either.

We counted our blessings. Geo was well. The children were doing well. We had a new home—no more shoveling snow, no more flooded basements. What could be better than that?

And after what we'd been through, how bad could the future be?

It took only a week to find out. Jim was in a terrible automobile accident, the force of the collision catapulting him from the front seat through the rear hatchback and onto the pavement. He suffered multiple lacerations and internal injuries. He required plastic surgery.

He lost eight teeth. It was remarkable that no bones were broken or that the glass he crashed through did not sever an artery or pierce an eye. When I saw him in the emergency room, his face a mass of clotted blood, he winked at me and said, "Hi, Pops, I'm sorry I smashed the car."

I never thought those words could sound so good.

We come now to Christmas, which after Jim's accident was more meaningful than usual and one we thought would be truly special. It was, but not for the right reasons. I woke up a few days before Christmas to the sound of rushing water, not too different from that of floods I had covered. I checked all the taps in the house, and they were fine. The noise seemed to get louder as I passed the front door, so I opened it and saw that the corridor had become a river about twelve inches deep. Funny time to install an indoor pool, I thought. I put on my boots and waded to the lobby.

In our old house we had worried about water coming up from the sewer. In our new house it was coming down from the ceiling. A pipe in the sprinkler system had cracked in the thirty-below-zero weather, and the sixteen thousand gallons in the reservoir were making their way to our door. Seventy units in the building, and the water chose ours to dump into. Carpets, wallpaper, furniture, clothing, books were ruined or damaged. What a mess!

It was a bleak Christmas, second only to 1968, when Geo was receiving radiation and her survival was anything but certain.

Geo: The dampness of the house aggravated some problems I'd been having for several months. I had severe headaches and dizzy spells that never seemed to end. I was dropping my food, my eyeglasses, my pen. I fell out of bed.

It was easy to blame all of that on the flooding and dampness, the depression and exhaustion of cleaning up.

But I also had become terrified of driving because I
kept veering off the road—always to the right. I avoided
expressways and rush hours, and I wouldn't go more
than twenty-five miles an hour. I was in a state of panic,
wondering from day to day if I'd be confident enough to
drive and afraid of losing the independence my car
gave me.

I found myself avoiding close friends because I'd
begun stuttering, and I was feeling lonely.

I blamed everything on the flood, but I also had
another scapegoat. I was coming up on my fiftieth
birthday and told myself these things probably happened to everyone at that age. Maybe that's why fifty is
such a dreaded birthday, I told myself—everything
falls apart.

I ran out of excuses one day when I had a seizure,
found myself propelled out of the kitchen to our en-
trance hall where the carpet had been removed, and I
gashed my head on the concrete floor. It swelled up and
bled profusely. I could not ignore that or charge it up to
a "mid-life crisis." I went to my doctor, who patched it
up and told me to see a neurologist.

When Bud and I walked into his office, he looked at
me as though I didn't belong there. He said I looked too
healthy, but when I couldn't stand on one leg without
falling or walk a straight line, he (and nine residents in
his office) agreed that something was wrong.

He scheduled a number of tests. The next day, for the
first time in seven years and with many misgivings, I
was to check into the hospital.

It was completely unexpected. I'd had no time to
prepare; the house was still a mess. But most of all, I
was concerned about the children. I knew they could
take care of themselves (they were twenty-one and
eighteen then), but I wondered how they would manage
emotionally.

A few days later I found myself strapped into a Magnetic Resonance Imager (MRI), which harnesses magnetic and radio waves to detect abnormal hydrogen and

proton reactions in the body. The test itself was not painful, but the huge machine, which produces a magnetic field forty thousand times that of the Earth's, was frightening and claustrophobic. I was told not to move or even breathe deeply. The technicians left the room, and I was isolated, except for Bud, who had asked to stay with me. I lay perfectly still for almost an hour, the machine making a terrible rat-a-tat noise that Bud likened to fifty-caliber machine guns he'd been around in the army.

The results of the scan, which were available within minutes, showed an enormous cyst affixed to the base of my brain. The pictures were so clear that even Bud and I could recognize the cyst that covered the back of my head, ear to ear.

There was only one way to remove it: brain surgery that would take place in four days. What an irony! I, who had faced cancer squarely, had never been able to imagine how people handled the terrifying news that they needed brain or open-heart surgery. It was awesome! All kinds of terrible fantasies clouded my thinking when I was alone. Fortunately that happened only at night, as family, friends, and hospital personnel I'd gotten to know in my many hospitalizations over the years dropped by and kept me occupied during the day.

I prayed an awful lot, zipping off to the chapel several times a day. That was another thing that frightened me. What if I wouldn't be able to walk, or drive again? I knew that was certainly a possibility. What about talking? The worst blow to a communicator is not to be able to communicate.

I had kept my promise to God and had tried to be "Super Coper." I had cared for my husband and children, I had never wavered from my faith, I'd kept my sense of humor which had always kept us going, and I had never asked, "Hey, God. Why me?" I had done my best and had even endured all the pain without complaint. And now I found myself asking, "Is this fair?"

The brain surgery was terrifying and the riskiest I'd

ever faced. It wasn't like removing a breast. I was afraid that the slightest slip of the scalpel, or going deeper into the brain than originally planned, would permanently affect my motor coordination, speech process, and the memory I take so much pride in.

It wasn't simply a matter of surviving the surgery. How would I survive *after* the surgery? Would the tumor be malignant? Would I be an invalid? Would it change what was me forever? There were so many implications to worry about. What if I came through the surgery and *didn't even know it???*

Bud: There comes a time when pain is so great you simply stop feeling it.

I remember being injured in a pickup game of basketball when I was in college. I was in the air, bringing down a rebound, my elbows pointing downward, when someone hit me from behind, slamming me hard to the floor, elbows first. I've never felt so much pain, and for weeks afterward I hurt so much I was barely able to move my arms even to brush my teeth or to dress myself. But within a few minutes after that injury I had resumed playing because I didn't feel anything. I was numb.

Emotional pain can be as excruciating as physical pain, and I was numb, too, on the day Geo had brain surgery.

My mother and uncle, Mike Savoy, came to the hospital that morning, and we all walked alongside Geo as she was wheeled to the operating room. We were no comfort to her or to each other. Geo, facing the riskiest surgery of her life, was laughing, joking, smiling, trying to cheer us up, as though she were on her way to a manicurist instead of a neurosurgeon.

Several friends came by that morning. Geo had asked them to look after me. We talked about everything except Geo's surgery—sports, politics, business—as though nothing else was going on.

I didn't return to Earth until the surgeon found me

wandering around several hours later. All feeling returned when he told me the surgery had gone well. He had drained the massive arachnoid cyst at the base of her brain. There was no malignancy. Geo would be fine.

I hugged my mother and realized the other people in the surgical lounge—total strangers until that morning—were cheering. I was so happy I didn't even shed tears of relief.

Later that afternoon, when Lou Pagones, my closest boyhood friend, unexpectedly came by, I finally broke down. When I told him Geo was going to be all right, he broke into tears and embraced me. There we were: two middle-aged men hugging each other and crying together. I'm glad no one had a camera.

Geo: My brain surgery was on February 2, 1984. Miraculously, the huge cyst was benign. A permanent shunt was implanted to drain fluid into my spinal column.

About the only thing I remember in intensive care was that on Saturday night (the surgery had taken place Thursday), I drove the nurses crazy begging for a telephone. They kept ignoring me because they thought I was still out of it. But Kerry was going to her first school dance, and Bud had gone home to see her off. I was disappointed that I wouldn't be there when her date came to pick her up. She had wanted to cancel it before my surgery, but I had begged her not to. After I kept banging on the bed and screaming, the nurses brought me a telephone so that I'd quit disturbing the other patients.

When I dialed home, Bud answered the phone, shocked to hear my voice. To our further disappointment, Kerry had already left, and I didn't get to tell her I was well. This bothered me because I wanted to be sure that the children both knew that I was going to be okay and that intensive care was routine procedure for brain surgery patients. Another reason for my concern about Kerry was that her favorite teacher, a young

woman of thirty-two, had collapsed in class the week
before, from a brain tumor. She was one person Kerry
would have turned to for support.

The first thing I did when I left intensive care was to
thank God that I had survived the surgery so well and
there was no malignancy.

The second thing I did was to put on my favorite wig,
and—presto—I looked like myself again. In fact, some
people thought I'd simply had a surface cyst or tumor
removed—no big deal. Others told me I made brain
surgery look so easy, like one of those television com-
mercials for outpatient clinics.

I recuperated remarkably well, eager to be in charge
of myself again and looking forward to going home. I
felt I could do everything I'd been able to do before
surgery, maybe even better.

Within a week after surgery I felt great. The night
before I was scheduled to be released, close friends
brought pizza to my room. I'd been craving it, and they
brought it as a reward for my having recovered so well.

The celebration was premature.

The following day (ten days after surgery) I contracted meningitis. The pain was the worst I'd ever
experienced. Pain medication brought no relief. I was
hooked into a battery of intravenous medications and
felt I was being kept prisoner in my bed. My speech was
so slurred no one could understand me. I lost all motor
coordination. I got very angry. I even hallucinated, so
that there were moments when I didn't seem to know
what was going on.

One moment I was well on my way to recovery, the
next I was sicker than ever before and had to fight
harder than ever to get well again. While we were
relieved that I did not have cancer again, we realized
that I did have a life-threatening problem, one that took
much to deal with and recover from.

Bud: The meningitis was like a kick in the groin, like

being blindsided after the whistle had blown. One day Geo was almost totally recovered; the next she was sicker than ever and fighting for her life.

I never had seen her in such pain, even after her mastectomies and hysterectomy, and for the first time I saw her unable to monitor her own treatment or to understand, much less control, what was happening to her.

When she left the hospital, she could not walk or even stand. Her speech was so slurred I could not understand her, and I was afraid she might never return to normal.

For months she could not move without assistance. Even though her memory and thinking were crystal-clear, she had almost no motor coordination and had to be fed and bathed. She was in great pain, and her head spun with every movement. Her features were distorted by the steroids she was taking to help reduce the swelling of the brain.

Whatever improvement I was able to see was measurable only in micro-millimeters. I'm convinced that only her faith and fierce will to live pulled her through.

Geo: My faith in God has sustained me all my life, and I trusted my neurosurgeon who kept assuring me that I would get better. I wanted so much to believe that. I've gone through every adversity and operation believing that I would recover quickly and be stronger than ever before.

I've always been an optimist. I don't know if this is a trait you are born with or develop later in life, but I consider it my strongest asset. My doctors have repeatedly told me that this attitude has helped me greatly in fighting cancer.

People who visited me in the hospital told me that if anyone could handle brain surgery and survive it with a smile, I could. Lucky me!

When I was finally discharged, my mom came in from Tulsa to be with me. I hadn't wanted her to see me in the hospital, with tubes all over and my speech slurred, because I thought she would be devastated. I suppose all mothers would, seeing their "baby" in such distress.

But I hadn't counted on how tough things would be at home. I needed her for everything: to move about the house, to get in and out of the tub, for my meals, for housework. She was an enormous help, but I know she often cried because she could not do more and because my condition brought her heartbreak. Mom stayed for over a month and was emotionally exhausted. Although I still needed help, she needed rest, so she returned to her home, feeling guilty because I was so ill. I, on the other hand, kept reassuring her that I was doing much better. We both tried to convince each other that the worst possible crisis had been surpassed and that our lives would soon return to normal.

But they didn't.

Shortly after she returned to her home in Tulsa, torrential rains over the Memorial Day weekend caused widespread flooding and knocked out electrical power and telephone lines. Water began rising in their home, and as they tried to go outside, lightning struck and set their house on fire. Within seconds the flames leaped fifty feet into the ugly sky.

Nearly overcome by smoke, they ran out but were trapped by angry, swirling waters that carried off everything that wasn't anchored. Clinging desperately to a porch railing, they watched in horror and wondered whether they would drown or perish from the intense fire that was consuming more than seventy years of their lives' work, memories, and personal belongings.

Miraculously, people in a motorboat rescued them seconds before their flaming house collapsed.

I couldn't imagine their painful thoughts as they witnessed the devastation. My Uncle George lost irreplaceable religious items—vestments, relics, books, etc.—from his fifty years in the priesthood, and my mother even lost her wedding band.

Everything that had had meaning in their lives was gone.

It was one of life's unbearable moments. They had survived a harrowing experience and needed time to grieve over their loss much as someone who has experienced loss from illness. I was relieved they weren't immobilized by depression or self-pity.

On the contrary, they were able to come to terms with the fact that things never would be the same and were ready to rebuild from scratch using nothing more than memories and determination.

I wanted desperately to be with them, but, forbidden by my doctors to fly, I had to be content for the moment to send money, clothing, and other things they would need and to telephone words of encouragement. We were deeply moved by help that was extended to them from other parts of the country, particularly from parishes my uncle had served as pastor. Just as my mother's presence helped me recover from surgery, the outpouring of help and comfort from friends helped Mom and Uncle George recover from their loss.

This terrible episode reconfirmed that waiting for things to be settled just right was futile. Things never would be perfect. But as long as there was love and support, we could survive anything that came our way.

After I finally was able to fly down to see them, I felt tremendous gratitude that I had inherited some of their spirit and appreciation for life. That probably had enabled me to cope with so much illness and adversity.

But you know what? I don't know that I could have rebounded from their dilemma as they did.

Mine seemed easier to bear.

Bud: Coming home after forty-two days in the hospital was the best thing for Geo. There is a condition called *hospital psychosis* that often sets in when one has been hospitalized for a long period. No matter how good the care, the environment works against recovery. Going home marks the transition between being sick and getting well.

The most important part of her recovery was time.

Once she was taken off steroids her speech became less slurred and her motor functions improved. Her progress was slow but visible. It took many months and was very difficult, for her and for all of us, but eventually she did get well.

She pushed herself, as always, ordering her body to do the things she wanted it to do. At the same time she took charge of the tedious task of filing insurance claims for all the things that had been damaged by the flooding. I was certain then that she was going to be all right. Nobody I know fills out insurance forms just for fun.

People who didn't know refused to believe she had been so sick. Once, while taking a swimming course to help rebuild her strength and agility, she was chastised for not venturing to the center of the pool with the class.

"I can't," she said. "I've had brain surgery and lose my balance easily."

"Sure," her instructor said. "That's the best excuse I've ever heard in all my years of teaching!"

3
Cancer Is a
Family Disease

Bud: There is a story about a Frenchman who was asked what he did during the French Revolution.

"I survived," he said.

Often, when I think of the battle my wife has had with cancer for the last twenty years, I feel the same way, for in its pain and upheaval it has been a revolution, changing our lives permanently.

Georgia is something of a walking miracle, having overcome a devastating prognosis to become a recognized authority in the area of emotional rehabilitation of patients with life-threatening and chronic illnesses, but I cannot think of her fight against cancer without breaking into tears.

I know that she has undergone the surgeries, that she has suffered the pain, that she has faced death more than once, and that I have experienced none of this, but I have scars just the same. So do our children.

When cancer strikes one member of the family, it strikes them all.

To some extent, writing this chapter has meant reliving it—not the happiest of tasks. But we think our experience may help healthy readers gain some understanding of the impact of critical illness on a family. And we hope our readers struggling with similar issues will know they are not alone.

HUSBAND, PROVIDER: BUD'S STRUGGLE

Bud: Georgia often has been asked why I did not leave her, a question I find in the poorest of taste and one that assumes people will walk away from their marriages and responsibilities as soon as the going gets tough. There are, unarguably, people who do that, but I believe most of us stick hard times out, not only hanging around but doing everything possible to overcome adversity in whatever form it appears.

Standing by a loved one in a time of illness or other crisis is simply something one should do. It may be hard. It may be expensive. But should one do less? The question never occurred to me, and quite frankly, I have resented its being posed by others, even when they mean it as an expression of compassion or concern. Do we not believe our marriage vows? Do we not stand by our commitments? Is it so hard to believe that people who love each other will stand by each other?

Commitment, however, does not make the going easy. A chronic illness, even if it is not immediately life-threatening, imposes a great number of hardships on a family, and when a life is on the line, those hardships grow at a quantum rate, multiplying and intensifying the pressures and tension on everyone.

Perhaps the most distinguishing thing about a long-term illness is that you spend more and more of your time dealing with it. Repeated trips to the hospital. Never-ending examinations, tests, x-rays. And every moment spent in a doctor's office is time taken away from the children, time taken away from teaching them, holding them, nurturing them. How many birthday parties can you postpone? How many parents' nights at school can you pass up?

How much of growing up can children miss? How much of watching your children growing up can you miss?

Geo's first hospitalization brought relatively few hardships to our house. Yes, there was fear. Yes, there was disruption. But it was confined mostly to explaining to young children why their mother wasn't going to be home for a couple of weeks and why she wouldn't be able to play with them when she returned.

Then, as she became weaker and sicker following her radiation treatments, we had to deal with the ever-more-obvious facts that she was not getting better and that both Mom and Dad were more worried than they had been a few weeks before.

As recurrences popped up and Geo had to reenter the hospital, explanations became not harder but impossible to offer. The children heard friends and relatives whisper about their mother. Sometimes they heard neighbors say things such as "She'll never come home again." They saw their father become moody, distant, unavailable, and they were sensitive enough to keep their distance, even though they undoubtedly needed more attention and coddling than ever before.

It was devastating enough for me to come to terms with the fact that my wife had an illness with an outrageously low cure rate, but dealing with the children, who either had sensed the gravity of her condition or had heard it in the whispers of adults around them, was something I couldn't handle.

How can you allay the fears of children who have been told, "Be good or your mother might not come home again" or "Your mother got sick because you weren't nice to her"? I was waiting for the same voices to tell me she got sick because I hadn't been a good enough husband.

Those were terrible days. Fear, frustration, and a
feeling of hopelessness filled every moment. As a boy I
had read of the ancient Spartans and had admired their
ability to face calamity without so much as a whimper.
My favorite part of the Bible was the book of Job, and
while I had vowed to face my own trials with equanim-
ity, strength, and courage, I suddenly found I was not as
brave as I wanted to be, and I was angry with myself
for being weak in a time of crisis.

There were two things that helped me cope. I always
have been a prayerful person, finding sustenance and
support in prayers, even if they are not always answered. Of course I prayed, perhaps with more fervor
than ever before. I prayed that Geo's life be spared, that
she be returned to health because the children needed
her and I needed her. But I prayed also for wisdom and
courage and strength to face whatever was coming.
Sometimes I think prayer is more a matter of reaching
within yourself than it is of asking God for help, but
whatever it is, I have found it a wonderful way to ease
anxiety and fear. (I'm not sure it helps baseball players
hit better, but then again, maybe .220 hitters need some
Divine intervention!)

The second thing that helped me was the way Geo
was responding to her illness. She was so brave, so
optimistic, so filled with cheer even as she battled her
physical pain, she made me feel better. If she could face
it with strength and courage, could I do anything less?

Geo: Living with cancer was no easy task for me. But
learning to live with my cancer was even more difficult
for my family, because few of them recognized what
they were facing. Bud thought, How can I feel sorry for
myself and complain when I'm not the one with the
pain?

However, his emotional pain, anger, stress, fear, anxiety, bewilderment, and feelings of helplessness were
sometimes more acute than mine. Few outsiders understood that when I suffered, he did too.

We learned that with everyone's attention focused on me, it was hard for my family to see their distress as normal.

Life-threatening illness weighs just as heavily on other relationships, such as a mother/daughter or mother/son who've been together their entire lives, sisters and brothers, best friends, live-ins. They've carved out a lifestyle around each other and cannot contemplate being left alone.

We've met spouses who tried to express their depression and exhaustion only to be admonished for thinking of themselves when the patient's well-being is what really matters.

"Jack" told me of the difficulties he experienced in keeping up with his wife, who suffered from a series of life-threatening illnesses. He felt it was affecting him far more than it was her. The highs and lows, the sudden decisions regarding her care, made it nearly impossible for him to concentrate on his work. He didn't know which required precedence: his job, which also provided the medical benefits, or his wife's illness.

Our situation was similar. But because I am basically an optimist, I plunged right in and tried to make up for lost time. However, this made it more difficult for Bud. He experienced the pain and illness secondhand; consequently, his needs and feelings weren't usually considered by those around him. He wasn't excused from performing his normal duties and responsibilities as readily as I was. The demands of his job, our house, and our family didn't go away just because I needed extra attention.

It distressed me to see my husband under such a strain. I constantly tried to cheer him up and convince him that I was feeling great and doing well. Then suddenly, a new complication would intensify his concern.

Bud's work was very demanding. A very private person, he relaxed by reading and listening to opera. I knew it was very important that he do things that bring him peace and pleasure to the degree that he could while preoccupied with worry.

I got firsthand experience with his perspective when I was suddenly cast in the role of spouse instead of patient. Bud became ill.

One sunny Saturday afternoon while we were driving out to the country for a late lunch, Bud blacked out at the wheel. We had been enjoying an entire day to ourselves, relaxed, happy, chatting, when he seemed to go into a trance. He passed out, oblivious to the heavy fifty-mile-an-hour traffic around us. I thought he had died. I was terrified but didn't panic. By the grace of God, I brought the car to a safe halt and revived him. I realized later that if I hadn't responded as quickly as I did, we would've had a fatal accident.

Bud has never wavered from my side; now it was my turn to care for him.

As I waited for Bud to undergo an MRI (Magnetic Resonance Imager) scan, all my own ugly memories came flashing back. I had had the highly sophisticated test twice and had gotten bad news in both instances. It seemed highly implausible that both Bud and I would have a cyst or tumor in the brain. I wondered if he understood the reason the doctor wanted him to have this scan. I wanted so badly to talk with him about it, but I couldn't force myself to come right out and ask him.

Suddenly there was a barrier between us; I found I was withholding full expression of my anxiety and fears so as not to alarm him.

The part of our relationship I treasure most is being so close and so supportive of each other; consequently, I felt more alone with my burden of worry. Here was another crisis in our lives and I was forced into sudden isolation. I was concentrating hard and was constantly occupied with trying to sort out what I should or could share with Bud.

This, I realized, is what it means to be the spouse of

someone who is ill. No matter how close you are or how much you want to share, you can't let it all hang out anymore.

The initial tests were inconclusive, so his doctors placed him on medication and ordered him not to drive, and I became his primary chauffeur. This was ironic because, since my brain surgery in 1984, there are days when I'm unable to drive because of lack of motor coordination. For over a month Bud relied on my driving him to his doctors, the hospital, to work, and wherever else he wanted to go. What a role reversal for us!

I don't know how this situation can be made easier. It's hard to respond to others, even those in situations that parallel ours, because we don't have a magic solution.

I do know, though, that I could never have endured what I've had to without my husband at my side, for he is my source of strength. In return, he tells me that he couldn't have survived it without someone like me, who has handled it as I have.

Bud: Geo's illness had a profound impact on my work. I suppose that it matters little whether one is an athlete or an astronaut; it is difficult to concentrate on your job when a loved one's life has been threatened. Repeated absences from work don't help one's career, either.

In the three years immediately preceding Geo's first bout with cancer I had been involved to some extent in our coverage of most of the important stories of the time, sometimes as the primary reporter, sometimes in a backup or supportive role—space shots, the Richard Speck murders, political conventions, campaigns, and riots, to name a few.

My first major assignment when I returned to work following Geo's first mastectomy was to produce our election-night coverage of General Curtis Le May, the former commander of the Strategic Air Command, who was running for vice president on a ticket headed by Alabama governor George Wallace. But Georgia was

undergoing her radiation treatments during that time
and, realizing how debilitating they were, I knew I
could not be gone from home, so I asked to be removed
from that assignment. My superiors in New York were
very sympathetic, and I was assigned instead to help
coordinate the election-night coverage from our studios
in Chicago.

I was scheduled to help produce a space shot from
NASA headquarters at Houston not long afterward and
needed to be excused from that also.

I realized I probably never again would be able to
perform my job as I had before. I also began to worry
that my usefulness to the company had diminished and
that any ambitions I might have held were about to fly
out the window. I won't pretend that didn't bother me,
but a lot more was at stake than my ambitions, which,
after all, were not nearly as important as Geo's life and
the survival of our family.

I volunteered for another job within our bureau that
required less traveling. I figured that when Geo recovered I could always go back to what I had been doing. It
didn't quite work out that way.

Things never returned to even a semblance of what
they had been before cancer.

I was preoccupied with Georgia's condition, so much
so that I found it hard to concentrate on my work. It
seemed as though almost every minute of every day was
spent worrying about her, wondering if she would survive and terrified she might not. I noticed most of the
people I worked with kept their distance from me, and I
thought at first it was because I was displaying a less-
than-cheerful demeanor. I realized much later they
simply didn't know what to say to me, and I understand
that, but at the time, their aloofness caused me considerable pain. I needed someone to talk with, and there
was no one.

That was hard to take, but almost as hard was my
self-imposed grounding. There is hardly anything more

important to a journalist than to be on the scene of a major story. True, I was kept busy at the office, working long hours putting together stories that were shipped in or transmitted electronically, writing and narrating reports for our various newscasts and syndication, but I missed being where the action was.

In May of 1970, for example, four students were killed by National Guardsmen during a Viet Nam War protest at Kent State University in Ohio. It was one of the biggest stories of the year, one of the biggest stories of the war, and I had to watch it on television.

Please understand, I know the story is much more important than who covers it; the lives of those four students, their families, and others affected by their deaths are infinitely more important. But it is the sad task of journalists to report stories such as this. I felt I should have been there, and I was upset that I wasn't.

I missed many stories over the years, and I watched a number of people pass me up on that mythical ladder of success. I, however, was measuring success in other terms: Geo was alive, we were taking care of the children, we were paying our medical bills, and we were working to help other cancer patients.

In the seventies expansion hit television news. Fifteen-minute news shows became thirty-minute shows. New programs were added to the daily schedules of networks and local stations alike. Newsrooms stayed open around the clock. The Watergate episode stimulated the public's interest in political events, and the rediscovery of "investigative reporting" inspired thousands of college students to enroll in journalism schools. We were a booming business, and I, along with almost everyone else in it, became busier than ever, routinely putting in fifteen-hour days. I was getting more time on the air, particularly on "Good Morning America," and I was happy to once again be doing something that was professionally and personally satisfying. Nevertheless, I was troubled.

Perhaps someone whose life has not been threatened or whose family enjoys good health can accept the long hours and other demands of his or her career, sacrificing part of the present in order to build for the future. The present, though, is all we can count on, and every day I wondered if I was wasting it.

It was as though I had to decide what was more important—making enough money to pay our bills, especially our medically related bills, which were draining us, retaining my own sanity by doing a job I liked, or finding another, less demanding job that might not pay as well and might not include Geo on an insurance plan. The possibility of losing insurance coverage was unthinkable. I stayed where I was.

I'm convinced it was the right thing to do. That kind of decision is faced daily by families living with debilitating and costly illnesses that require—no, demand—sacrifices by all. The strength to make tough decisions comes from their love and willingness to share all problems.

When you've got that, living with decisions is easy.

THE CHILDREN: JIM'S STORY

Geo: Serious illness in a family can be traumatic for adults, but for children, who can sense that something is wrong even if they don't know what it is, it can be devastating. Our children were very young when I first became ill. Bud and I did our best to help them understand what was happening, for we believe that any crisis is more manageable if information is shared as problems arise.

We wanted our children to avoid permanent scarring and encouraged them to vent any feelings of resentment or anger. We tried to be alert to their reactions even when they seemed indifferent or were too young to understand. Ignorance does not shield children from hurt; it only makes them more vulnerable.

We felt the important thing was to communicate with our children and to tell them exactly what was happening to their lives and the lives of their parents.

We always had tried to be honest. We had treated their adoption openly and talked with them about it in the hope that it would not become an issue later in their lives. Similarly, we chose to be honest about my illness, telling them that my life had been threatened. We felt it was better to handle it this way than to pretend everything was all right. I think we made the right decision, but that doesn't mean we didn't have problems.

Jimmy was five years old and in the first grade when cancer disrupted our happy household. He had always been an active, friendly, and precocious youngster who could read at four, but my illness turned him into an anxious, scared little boy. He told me once that he left for school every morning wondering if I would still be alive when he got home.

He became restless and fidgety in class, unable to concentrate. His teachers, and even our pediatricians, failed to recognize his fears. Instead of helping him, some of them made matters worse by scolding him, punishing him, even suggesting to him that my condition would worsen if he didn't start paying attention and doing his work. Jim was deeply depressed, and no one recognized it.

This pattern followed him everywhere—school, Cub Scouts, church. People who seemed to believe that cancer was a punishment, kept telling him never to displease or disobey me because I would become sick and have to return to the hospital again, a fact we did not learn until many years later, after untold damage had been done.

Since I was hospitalized more than thirty times, Jim must have had the weight of the world on his small shoulders, when all he yearned for was to be a carefree kid.

Looking back, we see that Jimmy's behavior had a

consistent pattern. If I was in the hospital, Jim would
not produce or participate in class. If I was home, he'd
bring me a one hundred every day. He, as all children,
needed a sense of security and needed to know that all
was well in his world.

Kerry, on the other hand, was only two-and-a-half
and, as she told me many years later, didn't know that
what was going on around her was unusual. She was a
beautiful baby, easy to love and very cuddly. People
liked to take care of her because she was so easygoing,
with none of the fears Jimmy had or the problems they
brought him. Kerry's shyness made them approach her
in a gentle way so that she would respond.

As she grew older and began to understand what was
happening, she changed very little. She was always
pleasant and eager to please. We had to remind her
from time to time that it was okay to express an opinion
or to say no once in a while. She did her homework. She
got high grades. She helped around the house. She
wrote me loving letters. Kerry, in fact, reacted to my
illness in exactly the opposite way that Jim did.

Maybe that's because it's the oldest child in a family
who usually inherits responsibility. That certainly was
true for Jim, and it was thrust upon him at an age when
he should have been more concerned about looking for
worms or chasing dogs around the block. Even when I
was not in the hospital, doctors' appointments often
kept me away from home until late afternoon, so Jim
had to look after his sister, remember whose house they
were going to for lunch and where they were going
after school. Many times he missed playing with his
friends during school holidays because I needed him
with me to watch Kerry.

You have to remember that these were not isolated
incidents; they were a way of life. The children were at
an age when they needed supervision and care, and I
was either hospitalized or following a pressing schedule of medical treatments that left me so exhausted that
I was not able to provide either.

We were blessed with many friends who were concerned, understanding, and sympathetic, but no matter how much they helped us it wasn't enough. There seemed to be no end to our need for baby-sitters or rides, and although our friends were extremely generous with their time and assistance, they had their own responsibilities; sooner or later, they got tired of helping. Enough, after all, is enough, and as I went through surgeries and recurrences, seemingly without end, we recognized that our friendships were being strained.

I was in the hospital again when Jim entered high school, and again he didn't do any work. His fears about my health intensified greatly, but he didn't say that. Instead, he abruptly announced that he wanted to look for his birth-mother. I could understand his desire to find her because I also would want to if I had been adopted, but the way he dumped it on us upset me deeply. I felt rejected and, consequently, hurt. Bud was furious, interpreting Jim's concern as an act of rebellion that increased the level of turmoil in our house and created another problem that had to be dealt with.

Jim's search came to an abrupt end when the adoption agency could not give us any information we did not already have, and that tore him apart. "I've lost one mother," he told me, "and it looks like I'm going to lose you too when you die. I have to have someone to hang on to." He ran away, leaving behind a note telling us not to look for him. It was signed, "Jim, last name unknown."

As much as that note hurt, it told us how much Jim was suffering, made us understand how deeply my illness was affecting him, and further emphasized the treacherous path cancer cuts through a family's soul. (Jim told us several years later that he never would have brought up the question had he not been so afraid and insecure at that time.)

Jim had sold his watch and bicycle and used the money to buy a bus ticket to Kansas City, where Bud's sister, Demi, lived. She called to tell us he arrived there. He stayed for a week, and then Bud drove down to pick him up, using the ten-hour drive back as a time to talk things over. Father and son seemed to come to an understanding, but Bud could not promise that my health would improve, and Jim could not be expected to overcome his fears by the time he got home.

He continued to rebel, not in a destructive way, but by breaking curfew, not doing his homework, and generally being a pain.

When others—friends, relatives, teachers, priests—tried to talk to Jim, they managed only to make things worse. One police captain, not knowing he was adopted, told Jim to stop making trouble for his courageous mother who had given birth to him and who was now fighting for her life. The poor man succeeded only in exacerbating the situation.

It was during this period of time that I had the hysterectomy and was going through a very rough emotional period caused by the menopause that had been purposely induced in an effort to curtail the production of hormones the doctors thought were causing the recurrences of cancer. I had crying spells and horrendous bouts of depression, intense hot flashes and sudden freezes. Because the doctors were trying to eliminate the hormones in my system, they could not, of course, administer traditional hormone therapy to help me. It was a physically painful and emotionally anguished time in my life.

We needed a respite. We needed time to heal, time to deal with my physical problems and with the way the illness was straining our family bonds, but we didn't get it.

We tried counseling through the Family Guidance Center at the hospital at which I received my treatment. But at this point it only made things worse. There was time in each session to pour out things that made each of us hurt, then we had to leave, taking our own hurt with us and, worse, taking everyone else's hurt home for a week until it was time to return and pick up where we left off.

I think we wanted an instant solution. Unfortunately, it doesn't exist. The counselor told us things probably would get worse before they got better.

We eventually stopped going together. Bud had always confided in me and didn't like the idea of a third party involved in our problems; Jimmy simply stopped showing up. But I continued my counseling sessions and found them to be very beneficial.

Then Jim developed hypoglycemia and lost about twenty pounds as he grew about six inches. Hypoglycemia can be controlled by diet but he purposely ate all the things the doctor said he had to avoid, and even though, to our knowledge, he did not drink or smoke, as soon as the doctor told him he could not do so, he started drinking and smoking.

His condition became worse, and we were told he was bent on self-destruction. He dropped out of high school, and we found it difficult to be civil to him. Bud could barely concentrate at work, and I felt myself becoming sicker and weaker. I could cope with cancer, but I couldn't handle Jim's problems.

Bud: We were bewildered, and so was Jim, who didn't know what to do with himself or for himself. He was as miserable as we were. He, in fact, took over our lives. It seemed that we did nothing but focus on Jim. We spent an inordinate amount of time dealing with his problems, canceling our own plans, missing church, weddings, parties. Geo even missed doctors' appointments.

None of this made a difference and probably served only to prolong Jim's period of difficulty.

We received plenty of advice: "Throw him out of the house." "Send him to military school." "Lie about his age and enlist him in the army." "Find his birth-mother and let her take care of him."

Jim heard these things, too, and became even more insecure. Undoubtedly our thinking was clouded by health problems, the high cost of medical care, which was straining our financial health, and the way Jim was acting out his fears.

Finally we did what we should have done at the beginning. We took a tough-love stance and didn't back off. We told him we loved him, that he was a permanent part of our family, that we needed him and would never abandon him.

He told us that he had terribly low self-esteem. He thought that whatever was troubling him was not normal, and that made him feel different from other kids.

We also explained that we had been unprepared to handle the pressures and uncertainty imposed upon us by Geo's illness, that we had made many regrettable mistakes, but that we were doing everything possible to save her life and preserve our family.

One thing more: we told him he had to control the behavior he could control and that we would help him with the things he could not, but it was time for him to face his problems and try to deal with them.

Things did not get better at once, and they did not all get better at the same time, but Jim returned to school, got his diploma, and even enrolled in college, although he didn't stay there long. He stopped his reckless behavior and started thinking about the future. As we write this he manages an optical lab in the Chicago area and is doing very well. Our regret is that we did not recognize his pain at an earlier stage and did not know how to deal with it effectively.

Geo: He needed love. He needed reassurance. He needed acceptance. And he needed them reinforced regularly.

Jim now feels good about himself, and we are able to talk about the things—good and bad—that we've been through. He is very caring, helpful and pleasant to be with. In fact, he has been helpful to others experiencing conflict over their adoptions and has provided valuable direction to younger kids in trouble. We are very proud of him.

He told me that "as a mother, you have been guilty of only two things, loving too much and trying too hard." I was impressed with how much Jim had grown to a mature awareness of what upset him, why it did, and which coping strategies would work well for him. It made me feel that our lectures, direction, and perseverance had penetrated.

When I had brain surgery in 1984, Jim was twenty-one, and he came to the hospital every day, sometimes two and three times a day. He said he wanted me to know how much he loved and needed me and that I would not have to worry about him again. When I was scheduled to go home on Valentine's Day, he bought twelve dozen croissants for the doctors, nurses, and aides, along with a note thanking them for taking care of me.

As it turned out, I developed meningitis and didn't get to go home for another three weeks. But everyone at the hospital seemed to be much more attentive after Jim brought the croissants!

A lecture I attended once really hit home. The speaker talked about home rules and priorities, those that could and should be reinforced and those that you could be flexible about. She described a tree as the foundation, the branches as rules to reinforce, and the leaves as things that were flexible—in other words, sometimes you do and sometimes you don't.

When I came home and mentioned this to Jim, he said, "I understand what she was talking about. The only thing you scold Kerry about is picking up her messy room. To me, that's a leaf. She always cleans it if we're having company. She's good, she obeys, she hasn't made waves or upset Dad and you like I have. In fact, you're lucky she didn't rebel when I was causing problems. You and Dad acted like you didn't have a life of your own. I really shook the branches. Doesn't Kerry's behavior count for something? Is it so important to scold over a leaf?"

I don't think I could have described it more eloquently myself.

4
From Tears to Triumphs

Geo: These days it's practically impossible to keep cancer patients from knowing their diagnosis unless they're willing participants in their own deception. Magazine articles, TV specials, newspaper stories routinely cover all aspects of the disease. Hospitals, health agencies, and doctors' offices are filled with pamphlets about prevention, diagnosis, and treatment. The subject seems hard to escape!

But not so long ago the picture was quite different. Cancer was called a "long, lingering illness," and many families tried to keep it a secret. When several of Bud's relatives, including his father, had cancer in the 1950s, the individual families were involved in schemes duplicitous enough to make the CIA envious, but their efforts were self-defeating and added greatly to the tension already in the house.

The families thought that the patients didn't know. The patients thought the families didn't know. People spoke in whispers or seldom spoke at all. It was an

61

elaborate scheme in which people succeeded only in fooling themselves.

I decided then that if ever I had a serious illness, I did not want it kept secret from me. I wanted to know. Now, after all the years of stress, I can't begin to imagine what the emotional atmosphere of our home might have been if I had been lied to or if we had chosen not to tell our family and friends.

Yet even as I was recuperating, some people tried to talk me into believing I hadn't had surgery for breast cancer. "It's probably just a cyst." "Maybe they made a mistake." One would have to be impossibly stupid to fall for that, but I think people were so afraid to say the word *cancer*, so unwilling to accept its existence, and so fearful it could happen to them, they simply denied it in any way they could.

Nevertheless, my openness and my insistence on putting on a happy face struck a chord with many, and almost immediately people began calling me to talk about our mutual problem. Doctors asked me to talk with their patients. Men approached Bud, for the first time, they said, to unload suppressed feelings about their wives' illness.

All of that gave me an idea of how I could keep that promise I'd made to God: to help as many sick and despairing people as I could. I still had rough periods of my own to get through, but I used that time to compile a mental list of all the things I would do if I were in charge. Since no one had articulated the needs of cancer patients (publicly, anyway), I used my own experiences to figure out what had to be done.

The most crucial issue, the one that had to be dealt with first, was the lack of information, support, and empathy. I began pushing out ideas like a popcorn machine, so charged with enthusiasm over what I was going to do as soon as I got the darn illness out of the way, it helped me focus on getting well.

So much needed to be done that I wasn't going to let a far-from-hopeful prognosis keep me from doing it. I didn't think about dying. I thought about changing the world. That may have been presumptuous, but it reinforced my optimism and kept me going.

In late 1968 and early 1969, when I received radiation treatments, the pain, anxiety, depression, and fear were so debilitating it took all the courage I had to make it from day to day. Other patients I observed or spoke with clearly felt the same way.

Because of the fear, anxiety, and distress it brings, cancer is not simply an enemy of the body; it is an enemy of the psyche as well. It attacks the emotions as it attacks the tissues, and often the damage to the patient's emotional well-being is more serious than the damage to the body. But in 1968, our opportunities to talk about this stress, to find ways of dealing with it, were practically nonexistent.

Fear and pain are not, as most office hours are, confined to a Monday-through-Friday, nine-to-five schedule. Although that's something like saying, "the sky is blue," not exactly a startling and revealing new truth, it took some people by surprise when I pointed out that, in the middle of the night when people were scared to death or on weekends and holidays when they were lonely and depressed, there was no one around to talk to.

A call to most social service agencies produced a recorded message asking them to call back on the next working day or no answer at all. This infuriated me.

Why, I asked myself, should patients have to face illness alone with no one but their emotionally exhausted families to talk to? The answer was as obvious as the question: they shouldn't.

There were hot lines for alcoholics, drug users, draft evaders. Abortion counseling was available by phone. Social security information was just a call away. There was even a green thumb hot line for gardeners. Why not for cancer patients, whose very lives were at stake and whose survival depended greatly on their own response to the illness and their willingness to fight it? I determined there should be a twenty-four-hour-a-day telephone support service for patients and their families.

No one knows more about how it feels to have cancer than a cancer patient. So it was only logical that recovered patients who had an awareness of their feelings and the ability to cope with their illness would be of great support to newly diagnosed patients and become living examples that cancer is not always a synonym for death.

I told myself, and I promised God, that if I made it through the radiation I would do everything I could to create that service.

The logical place to start was at the American Cancer Society, which already sponsored programs such as Reach to Recovery and ostomy and laryngectomy clubs. I proposed my idea when I was asked to share my battle with cancer at the Chicago Unit's Annual Meeting in September of 1971. I know I surprised them. I think they were expecting a simple "I've got cancer and I'm glad to be alive" presentation, but even though I challenged them to create more work for the staff and volunteers, the response was overwhelming. Before we could get started, however, we needed the support of the national office.

Four months later, in January 1972, at the American Cancer Society's national crusade kickoff at New Orleans, I delivered the same speech to more than a thousand health professionals, volunteers, and staff members from all over the country. They had gathered to learn about the latest developments in cancer research and support so that their fund-raising activities would be informed and inspired.

I told them, "You need more than a doctor when you're fighting cancer. You need someone to lean on, someone to talk with, someone who cares, someone who understands, someone who has not only walked in your shoes but who is still around leaving footprints."

Although I had been told that the society was a conservative organization that needed time to digest new ideas, the response once again was overwhelming. I received a standing ovation, and delegates promised their support before they went home to tell their units what I had proposed.

My appearances on both occasions were so well received that they were fully reported in the newspapers and shown on television news broadcasts. I was invited to appear on TV and radio talk shows around the nation, and each one generated more invitations. I was astonished. After all, I was talking about cancer, a subject that had been a closet disease for so long. Nobody wanted to talk about it, hear about it, learn about it, yet suddenly someone was speaking out, someone who was not a movie star, a sports hero, or, like Yul Brynner, someone who had died of cancer and was speaking to us from the grave through antismoking television announcements he'd made prior to his death.

I think audiences related to me because I was not anyone famous, I was not wealthy, I did not have an ax to grind, and I wasn't asking for money. More importantly, I was not afraid to talk about cancer. Many, many other patients were tired of the silence and ignorance that surrounded the disease. Perhaps, through me, they were having their say.

Whatever the reason, I received mountains of mail and so many invitations I couldn't keep up with them all, but wherever I did go I talked about the need for that patient-to-patient hot line. I was busier than ever—even busier than before I became ill, and I was very active then—but the busy season, I soon discovered, was just beginning.

Meanwhile, the Chicago Unit of the Illinois Division of the American Cancer Society had given me a grant of about $3,000 to develop the pilot service. It took about a year to put together what became Cancer Call-PAC. The letters in PAC meant People Against Cancer. Bud and I thought it was an appropriate acronym that would be remembered easily by patients who wanted to call.

We worked with a committee made up of recovered

cancer patients, a doctor, a nurse, a lawyer, a chaplain,
a representative of the phone company, and the owner
of a telephone answering service who had given us free
service in tribute to his young wife who had died of
cancer. This dedicated group of health professionals,
patients, and others worked diligently to establish
guidelines, plan training sessions, and practice role-
playing.

We recruited more than one hundred "listeners,"
many of whom could speak a foreign language so that
immigrants who had trouble with English could also
have someone to speak with.

Call-PAC began operating on June 26, 1973, helping
to meet a vast area of human need—emotional support
and understanding—that too long had been neglected
in the treatment of cancer. I felt this could be the beginning of the healing process for many patients and a
necessary adjunct to the overall treatment of the disease.

We trained our volunteers to listen first and talk
later. We connected patients with listeners who had the
same kind of cancer. We did not offer medical advice or
intrude on the doctor-patient relationship. We did offer
understanding and hope, pointed out services that were
available—hospital beds from the American Cancer
Society, nursing help from the Visiting Nurse Association—referred patients to free pastoral counseling
when they needed more help than we could provide. We
helped give direction that so often is the turning point
in one's decision not to give up the fight for life.

Making people aware of a new service or product is
difficult without paid promotion, but ACS policy for-
bids the purchase of advertising. We did, however, have
a program people needed and wanted, so a little free
promotion went a long way. We sent brochures and
posters to hospitals and asked that their social services
and pastoral care departments tell their patients about
our service and give them the phone number. We pre-

pared public service announcements for radio and television stations and asked that they run them. The American Cancer Society sent letters to its Chicago unit volunteers.

We held a news conference, and among those covering it was Chris Wallace, who later became the White House correspondent for NBC News but who was then a reporter for WBBM-TV, the CBS station in Chicago. Chris said that because Bud worked for ABC it seemed to be pretty much a "house story" for WLS, the ABC station, but he thought it was important enough for others to cover because the service was unique. Bud was unable to convince Chris that he'd had nothing to do with WLS's interest in the story. Newspapers and wire services also covered it. I appeared on a television talk show that morning, and the phones rang off the hook.

The power of the printed and spoken word is enormous, but I think the news spread so quickly because people were waiting for what we had put together.

Hundreds of people called in Call-PAC's first week. I was somewhat surprised by the volume but not by the nature of the calls. Here's a sampling:

A teenaged girl asked, "How can I show my mother I care even though I can't stand to help change her bandages?"

A man who had undergone a colostomy told of his anguish at being served dinner on a paper plate while others at the table ate off china. He wanted to know how to assure people that his illness wasn't contagious.

A young child wanted to know what he could do to help a parent with cancer.

Friends asked, "How can I convey I understand? What can I do to help?"

Some people called for help with their anxiety on the day they got their diagnoses.

Long-term patients asked, "What can you do on the days you just don't feel like living?" They weren't contemplating suicide; they were just looking for a way to get through one more of a long succession of bad days. We heard that question, or a variation of it, with agonizing frequency.

People were not asking for medical help. They wanted emotional support, someone to hold their hand for a few moments. The calls came from men and women, young people and old people, professionals and blue-collar workers. Although we never asked their names, most volunteered them along with other information that confirmed what we already knew: that the fear and turmoil of cancer cuts through all races, all backgrounds, all social and economic states, all people.

The response to Call-PAC underscored the regrettable fact that our social progress has been far outstripped by our scientific progress. Our awareness of and expansion of ways to rehabilitate people is far behind our ability to refurbish buildings and develop new technology. But one product of the technology, the telephone, can be an invaluable instrument in both urban and rural areas, and soon we were deluged with requests to help set up programs in other cities and states.

The committee responded by preparing a packet of information on the project—everything from recruitment to training, operational data, and evaluation criteria. Some units, particularly those in metropolitan areas (where anonymity of caller and listener is easily kept), adapted Call-PAC exactly as we designed it. Other communities used our screening and training advice for patient-to-patient visiting and preparing volunteer leaders. Health agencies representing other chronic diseases wanted practical suggestions for organizing the phone network.

The widespread interest demonstrated two things: (1) patients and their families needed more than medical management of the disease; and (2) many recovered patients and health care professionals wanted to help—all they needed was a vehicle for their concern.

Call-PAC matched patients under stress with willing, well-trained volunteers who could honestly say "I understand." The service won an American Cancer Society Merit Citation, both for its uniqueness and for its emphasis on volunteers rather than on paid staff.

Call-PAC's success brought more opportunities but also more challenges. That promise to God was one I took seriously, and whether or not my survival and recovery resulted from our prayers, my promise or His intervention (which I believe it was), I had made a commitment, and I knew I had to keep my part of the bargain. I had envisioned, at first, helping people in a small way, one on one—neighbors, friends, relatives. I had no idea I would be involved in projects that would reach so many. Apparently, God had much more in mind for me than I realized.

Two amazing things happened almost coincidentally with the inauguration of Call-PAC. A first-person story I had written that appeared in the *Chicago Tribune*'s *Sunday* magazine was syndicated nationally, and a five-part special series on my battle with cancer was shown on WLS-TV, the most-watched station in Chicago.

Suddenly I had become something of a celebrity. When I appeared on the late Bob Kennedy's morning talk show, "AM Chicago," the station received 126 calls in less than an hour from people who wanted to talk with me. I was able to talk with several on the air, but, of course, there was not nearly enough time to respond to everyone who called. Later that day, one of the show's producers called me at home to relay the names and numbers of people who had called in. "I've sorted them out according to site," he said. "These are breast," and he gave me the list. "These are lung . . . , etc."

At church, at the grocery store, at the hospital, on the street, I literally was besieged by people, some of whom said they wanted to congratulate me for my spirit or my work but followed that by saying, "I had a breast removed last month," or "My mother is sick," or "What's that number to call for help?"

Bud and I had done extensive research to set up Call-PAC, so by that time I had a rather firm grasp on the nature of the disease, modalities of treatment, where treatment was available, the state of research, agencies that provided help and/or information. Without meaning to, I became a one-woman counseling and referral service.

At home our phone rang constantly, and we had to add a phone. I even received calls from social service agencies that wanted me to talk with their "clients." A caseworker at the Illinois Department of Mental Health told me she had too heavy a caseload and asked me to visit some of her cancer patients at their homes. I told her I wasn't qualified to do that.

Even some high-priced psychologists asked me to talk with some of their patients. They didn't, however, offer to share their fees with me!

All of this told me that much more work needed to be done, and if no one else was doing it, I would. My ability to do it surprised me almost as much as the opportunity. I never expected to be appearing on television championing a cause.

I was asked to cohost a fund-raising telethon on an Omaha television station just across the Missouri River from Council Bluffs, Iowa, where I was born and raised. We had a reunion with friends there, and it felt like a hometown-girl-makes-good,-gets-cancer story.

I never dreamed I'd be asked to travel around the country to lecture. But the invitations seemed to come by the dozens, and almost all of my energy was directed toward bringing the urgent need for improved patient care into focus.

Urgent was the key word for me. Patients have no way of knowing if they will survive and, if they do, for how long. I plunged in because I didn't know how much time I might have to do this work, so I accepted every invitation and traveled across the country trying to reach professionals, patients, and everyone else within earshot.

EVERY MOMENT COUNTS

Bud: Geo's ability to reach people was exceeded only by her vitality. I always went with her, mostly because I didn't want her to travel alone, but most of the time I was asked to be on a program to talk about our relationship and how the illness affected a patient's spouse. I was healthy, and she was supposed to be sick, but I tired long before she did, and she overwhelmed me with her energy and stamina. We spent so much time on the road she began to call me ABC's contribution to the American Cancer Society because the company permitted me to take time off whenever we were invited somewhere.

Audiences often were astounded when they first saw her because she didn't look sick. She was pretty and vital; she smiled and laughed and displayed such optimism and cheerfulness that, had she not spoken of her illness, it was impossible even to guess she was a cancer patient.

The reason for that was simple. She never permitted herself to give in to her illness, to its effect on either her health or her appearance. When the treatments caused much of her hair to fall out, she put on a wig and made it look like her own hair. She refused to wear an old robe around the house or go out without makeup. I likened her to Billy Crystal's Fernando character, whose philosophy was "it doesn't matter if you feel good as long as you look good."

It was the other way around for her, though. Looking good made her feel good. Unfortunately, many people think about patients in caricature, expecting to see them bleeding and bandaged, on crutches or in wheelchairs. Once, when we were in Washington, D.C., an ambulance pulled up to the television station just as we walked in. "Oh," someone said, looking at the ambu-lance, "that must be the cancer patient who's the guest today. I wonder if she'll make it through the show."

I wanted to correct him immediately, but I waited, hoping to be able to see his expression when Georgia was introduced. I couldn't, but I bet he was shocked.

Her healthy appearance enabled her to convey the positive side of cancer—the chance of cure if caught early enough and the expectation of resuming a produc-tive life after treatment. She was able to reach a large and varied group of people, including patients and nonpatients, health care professionals, clergy, re-searchers, fund-raisers—in short, just about everyone who had anything to do with the fight against cancer.

I think perhaps she embarrassed some who might have thought they were involved in a hopeless cause, but she inspired many more, and we no sooner would return home than we began to receive letters from them, telling us how they planned to act on her ideas.

Georgia's efforts began to show results in ways neither of us expected. Hospitals, churches, and schools began to pay more attention to and explore new ways of providing emotional support. She spoke at health fairs and seminars, medical schools and associations, and clergy congresses.

The City Colleges of Chicago asked her to teach a course exploring the impact of cancer on patients and families. It was conducted not in a classroom but in a conference room at a hospital where, it was thought, the "students," all of whom were patients or relatives, to-gether with some nurses, administrators, and cha-plains, would be more at ease.

I think the best way to describe what happened is to quote from a sermon delivered by one of the chaplains.

"As the word got out that Georgia had founded a place where folks with cancer could get together to share concerns and find strength and comfort, the de-mand for such groups exploded.

"As ill and depressed as many were when they came, as they got together, they discovered resources they didn't know they had . . . fellowship, happiness, a sense of purpose, and a feeling of inclusion with a 'family' with whom they could candidly share their fears and hopes and rediscover a sense of worth and self-dignity."

Sessions were covered by NBC and ABC for use on the "NBC Nightly News" and "Good Morning America." The reaction was totally unexpected and so was something else. The colleges paid her for teaching the class. It was the first time she had received anything but expenses for any of her appearances. She would joke about that, saying, "If I'm being paid what I'm worth, I guess I'm not worth anything."

At the same time, though, some people were telling her, "I'd love to be your agent because when I look at you, I see cash registers ringing."

Her appeal was clear, and so was the reason. Stories about cancer patients such as Nat King Cole, Brian Piccolo, and John Wayne, for example, always ended with the hero's death—poignant, emotional stories, certainly, but filled with despair, offering audiences plenty to cry about, little to take hope in.

Georgia's message could not have been more different. Sure, she was sick; sure, she had pain; but, to quote her, she "was still leaving footprints," talking about hope, not despair, survival, not death, laughter, not tears.

She was such a hit on some shows that she was invited back, not as a cancer patient but simply as Georgia Photopulos. In the television business, producers with shows to book have a little network of their own, checking with fellow producers in other cities in their search for good guests.

"Georgia Photopulos," was the response from a producer at WLS.

"Who is she? What's her act?"

"She doesn't have an act. She's a cancer patient."

"You've got to be kidding!"

It was something to watch. I had been in the business since my discharge from the army after the Korean War and had hardly made a stir. But she, with no training and no experience, was knocking them dead, and she was talking about cancer, of all things.

Some of the shows she appeared on won awards. The WLS series, called "Every Moment Counts," won several. It ran on the early and late newscasts for five consecutive nights in May 1973. Anchorman John Drury wrote and reported the series. He and camera crews followed us around for several weeks, coming to our house to film us there, accompanying Geo on a visit to her oncologist, following her to church, to a Call-PAC workshop, and even to the hospital where she had her radiation. There she talked about how she had come to look upon the huge machinery as a friend that had helped save her life.

The film crews and editors, most of whom I had worked with at one time or another, did a marvelous job. Drury's pieces, relating how Geo had faced her illness with faith, courage, and cheerfulness, were almost poetry.

Many of our friends thought I had arranged the entire project, but I had nothing to do with it. In fact, I was stunned when Drury and WLS news director John Mies asked me if we'd be receptive to the idea.

Later, the entire series was redone as a thirty-minute special that aired on prime time.

And when John Drury accepted one of the several awards the series garnered, he took Geo with him, sharing the spotlight with her.

A gracious man is John Drury.

Geo's work attracted attention, as one person put it, at the highest levels. She received a letter of congratulation from President Richard Nixon, and Illinois senator Charles Percy inserted a magazine article about her into the *Congressional Record*. She was named Churchwoman of the Year by the Greek Orthodox Church and received a Jefferson Award for Humanitarian Service from the *Chicago Sun-Times*. The American Cancer Society bestowed on her their Spirit of Courage Award.

She became the only patient on the National Task Forces on Breast and Uterine Cancer of the American College of Obstetricians and Gynecologists (ACOG), helping to write a nontechnical pamphlet explaining illnesses of the breast and uterus that you may have read in your gynecologist's office.

After Betty Ford's mastectomy and a local TV personality's death from cancer, she received calls from the three major networks and four radio stations simultaneously asking for interviews.

She participated in the first National Conference on Cancer Control and the Behavioral Sciences at San Antonio, Texas, in January 1975, and her presentation was published along with those of distinguished physicians, psychiatrists, and sociologists in *Cancer: The Behavioral Dimensions* (New York: Raven Press, 1976.)

When Georgia finished her presentation, the discussion and response moderator, Dr. Godfrey Hochbaum, professor at the School of Public Health, University of North Carolina at Chapel Hill, stated: "As I was listening, it occurred to me that Mrs. Photopulos has really said almost everything or has touched on almost everything we have discussed. Somehow I think she has communicated these issues much more effectively than any statistics or research finding that I could cite. It may be that the one thing I learned is that we should not talk so much about how we can communicate what to whom, but how can we be more sensitive to the people with whom we want to communicate and discover what they want and need. Maybe we should turn around and look at the whole problem from the other side."

Now, some people may shrug and say, "So what?" But remember, she had had no experience in this field before she became a cancer patient. She had had no training and no professional impetus to do any of these things. She was, as she liked to say, "just a housewife from Farragut Avenue in Chicago," but she was causing a sensation.

In April 1975, Geo and I were called to Washington, D.C., to confer with the National Cancer Institute's Division of Cancer Control and Rehabilitation and the Office of Cancer Communications. Her role was to develop a training program for use at the newly established Comprehensive Cancer Centers. She created materials, then conducted workshops for the staff of prestigious medical centers, such as Memorial Sloan-Kettering in New York, M.D. Anderson in Texas, Mayo, Harvard, UCLA, Denver, and Duke University, to name a few.

She assisted with the establishment of the nationwide toll-free Cancer Information Service, whose phone number is 1-800-4-CANCER. This was mandated by the National Cancer Act of 1971, the landmark legislation that greatly expanded, coordinated, and intensified the nation's effort to conquer cancer through research, diagnosis, treatment, and continuing care for patients. She continues to serve as a consultant.

When Julie Nixon Eisenhower presented a framed copy of that act to the Illinois Division of the American Cancer Society in spring of 1972, Georgia was chosen to receive it symbolically on behalf of the American Cancer Society and all patients.

A top official at the National Cancer Institute described her as "one of the nation's leading experts on emotional rehabilitation of cancer patients."

Some things that happened were simply astounding. In January of 1976, Geo was in Washington, D.C., conducting a workshop for the National Cancer Institute. This was the first time that I hadn't gone with her; I had come down with a viral infection that literally knocked me out. So, Elaine Tarant, a good friend who frequently helped Geo, accompanied her.

The American Cancer Society, at the same time, was preparing for its annual crusade kickoff by holding a tea at the British Embassy. First Lady Betty Ford, who recently had had a mastectomy, was to be the guest of honor, but she was undergoing treatment and couldn't be there.

Guess who took her place?

The American Cancer Society asked Geo to fill in for the first lady, and the next day her picture was on the society page of the *Washington Star* showing her sipping tea with Lady Ramsbotham, the wife of the British ambassador. I didn't believe it until I saw the picture.

Not bad for a housewife from Farragut Avenue!

One thing she didn't get to do, though, was to attend the First International Congress on Patient Counseling, which was held in the Netherlands in 1976. She had been invited by the chief of psychiatry at Rotterdam University, Dr. M. Kazemier, who had heard her presentation at San Antonio the year before. She was the only layperson invited. We did not work for a government or private agency, and since we had no private practice of our own and no funds to draw on, we were unable to go. Dr. Kazemier said that because of her expertise, "It was of the utmost importance" that she deliver a paper there and even tried to obtain funds from his government to cover our expenses.

In the end, everyone told us they couldn't help because we were in a unique category. Although Georgia had expertise that was in demand, she was just a volunteer, and they couldn't appropriate funds for volunteers. Georgia was disappointed and, for the first time, dejected.

WHY NOT REACH FOR THE MOON?

Geo: Dejection lasts only about as long as you let it and frankly I didn't have time for it. Fighting cancer was enough of a problem; I didn't need to disperse my energy needlessly, and I certainly didn't want to waste my time moping about things I couldn't change.

Events in life have an inexorable force of their own,

and once they're in motion you have no choice but to go where they take you. Cancer had its momentum; so did the way I fought it. Bad things had come in torrents. Good things did, too.

In September of 1975 I received a phone call from Bill Bell, the creator and producer of "The Young and the Restless," the immensely popular daytime drama on CBS. He wanted the character Jennifer Brooks to undergo a mastectomy, and he wanted it portrayed as accurately as possible from presurgical fear through postsurgical anxiety. He asked me to write episodes for a segment depicting Jennifer's anxiety, anger, depression, hostility, and ultimate acceptance.

It was a new challenge. I never had done that before and didn't know anything about writing television scripts—setting up scenes, giving directions to the actors, weaving one segment into another—but I jumped at the chance, especially when Bill told me the sequence would reach millions of viewers and would be an opportunity to show not despair but hope, courage, and inspiration.

Bill is known for his meticulous research and insistence on honesty, and he wanted a powerful story about breast cancer integrated into the reality of the characters' lives, including the interaction of family, physicians, and friends.

With Bill's supervision and fine work by the actors, the sequence turned out to be exactly what we had hoped for—an accurate and honest portrayal of a woman's fight with breast cancer. I had no trouble with the dramatic elements; breast cancer is dramatic enough and needs no embellishment.

The audience responded with, I'm told, an enormous amount of mail, and the episodes won an Emmy for best individual serial sequence. The American Film Institute put Jennifer Brooks's breast cancer sequences together for use as a training film because of its important message to women, and the National Academy of

Television Arts and Sciences planned to show the scenes to research students and science reporters.

In May of 1978, we received the biggest thrill of all—an invitation to the White House. The postal service issued a postage stamp honoring Dr. George Papanicolaou, the developer of the Pap smear, which is named for him. Because of our work in the field of cancer support and because we are of Greek descent, we were invited to attend the reception for his widow on the day the stamp was issued.

We had to present our invitation to the marine officer at the North Portico, and he pronounced our name perfectly. *"Photopulos,* as in *Acropolis,"* he said. We were impressed. Hardly anyone pronounces our name correctly if we haven't met before. Now, when people ask me how it's pronounced, I can't resist the temptation to say, "Photopulos, as in Acropolis. That's the way they pronounced it at the White House."

We had refreshments in the State Dining Room and met First Lady Rosalynn Carter and Marvella Bayh, the wife of Indiana senator Birch Bayh and herself a cancer patient with whom I had appeared on several TV programs. Each displayed a genuine interest in my health and my work, and Mrs. Carter asked a White House photographer to take a picture of us with them. When we received it a week or so later, we were surprised to see that both she and the president had signed it.

As the children grew older and many of our hopes for them were becoming a reality and I was comfortable that I was honoring my commitment to help others cope, I decided to do something special for myself: to get my degree.

I enrolled at Northeastern Illinois University (in Chicago), and received my degree in communication in health education in December of 1982. It was another dream come true.

The degree program required an independent study

project. Again, my illness provided both challenge and opportunity. All my years of working with cancer patients made me, I thought, an expert on coping. Nonetheless, what I "knew" from experience was one thing, and what I, or any other interested professional, could objectively demonstrate was quite another.

So I set out to create a questionnaire that would allow me to document patient/family needs and coping strategies. The trick was to ask the right questions and ask them in such a way that I could rely on the answers. I was interested in how patients felt they had coped and in what or who had helped or hindered the process. I was confident that patients would be eager to share their experience if they knew they would be understood; further, those who had coping strengths might not realize their value.

I prepared the questionnaire, field-tested it, and revised it. Someday I'll administer the questionnaire to many patients of many backgrounds with many types of cancer. When I have done so, you can bet I'll publish the results. Such data are bound to enhance communication between patients and their caregivers and help them understand each other's strengths and weaknesses.

I also was working on a way to keep my wig from sliding and falling off. Don't laugh—I'm serious. Most people anchor their wigs to a full head of hair, but those with hair loss cannot. I had lost much of my hair during my treatment, and it never grew back fully. It doesn't bother me that I don't "put up a big front" like Dolly Parton—but my wig is something else. I would never go without one. It makes me feel better, it makes me look better, but keeping it on can be a problem even with spirit gum or adhesive strips, which are uncomfortable for people who have had brain surgery, chemotherapy, or radiation.

I worked on this for years, experimenting with various methods until I developed one that actually worked: four plump fiber-filled cushioned pads, (two for the temples, one for the crown and one for the nape of the neck) that customized over-the-counter, one-size-fits-all wigs.

They worked so well for me I was sure they'd help others, and I was able to patent them. It's exciting to appear before a patent examiner and to walk through the inventors' museum telling yourself you're now right there next to Cyrus McCormick, Thomas Edison, and the Velcro man.

Convinced that the pads would help a large number of men, women, and children, I tried to find someone to produce and market them, but I kept running into dead ends. I was talking therapeutic, and everyone else was talking cosmetic. They didn't want to talk about illness or hair loss, but about wearing wigs for fun and fashion. After years of hard work and running into dead ends in the business world, I finally found a manufacturer in New Jersey to produce them, but he was unable to market them successfully, so we decided to do it ourselves.

I approached the manager of one department store chain near the UCLA Medical Center in California (where many patients are treated) about carrying the pads in his millinery department. He arrogantly informed me that his elegant clientele didn't have the kinds of problems I had described. Then he turned and walked away.

I tried many hospital gift shops, believing that patients could purchase them when they went for their treatment, but the managers made statements to the effect that patients rarely shopped there, and they preferred to carry items that were attractive gifts for their family and friends to buy.

Another time when the manager of a wig boutique had asked me to introduce the pads at a store in Chicago's Loop and assist customers with their purchase, I jumped at the opportunity. It was a large chain with fifteen stores that sold an incredible number of wigs. Ads appeared in the Sunday newspapers along with a photograph of me, and signs were posted at all the entrances of the store inviting customers to meet me in the wig department. Unfortunately, the store manager had seen the ad and had revised the promotion before I arrived there.

All references to hair loss, illness, and cancer—the real purpose of the wig pads—had been deleted, as if I were in the store to help people buy wigs for fashion and fun. Later in the day the manager stopped by and introduced himself. He commented on my healthy appearance and said that he had changed the signs so they wouldn't be a threat to his "well" customers. He nudged me and said, "I think you should quit worrying about sick people and let them look out for themselves. Don't mention your illness and you'll get a lot further."

If I wouldn't have been tried for manslaughter, I would have pushed him down the escalator.

I can't say that we didn't hope to make a profit, but I was certain millions of patients would be helped. I wanted to make the pads available and to keep the cost affordable to those who needed them. Some of the large companies I asked to distribute them wanted to charge more for them than they did for the wigs, and I wanted no part of that.

I was in the midst of a dilemma: patients wanted the pads because they were a comfortable and much needed solution to wig slippage, and health professionals who saw them were eager to inform their patients that the pads were available, but I had trouble finding retail outlets to sell the pads: "Not enough room for markups." "Use cheaper, recycled fiberfill instead of virgin; then there's more room for profit."

I worked as a one-woman production line out of my home, again asking friends and relatives for help, and managed to get the pads introduced in eighteen states and Canada. One night Bud came home after a fourteen-hour day to find me sitting exactly where he had left me—at the table, sorting wig pads, counting out twenty thousand pieces to fill the largest order I was ever to receive. It was like sorting twenty thousand toothpicks into piles of four (because there were four pads to a set), a tedious, boring, and aggravating task. When I was still at it at midnight, Bud and the kids demanded that I stop, and I said, "You're right, I can't take this anymore," and threatened to jump into the reservoir near our home. Kerry laughed and said, "After what you've been through, don't do that over those lousy wig pads!"

I was exhausted, and it wasn't cancer that had worn me down. We had learned the hard way that without enormous sums of money it's awfully hard to get a new product on the market. We didn't have the money or know-how and experience, so after several years of trying, of being treated shabbily by large companies, some of whom tried to rip us off, we decided to put the venture aside, even though many years remained on the life of my patent.

That's when I decided to resume the writing I love to do, which allowed me to reach many more people. My first column ran in the Pulitzer newspaper chain in the Chicagoland area in June 1984, with access to over a million households. I began hearing from many patients, but, as we learned with Call-PAC, the letters from family members outnumbered those from patients. The column "Of Tears and Triumphs" was originally intended to address the fears and concerns of those living with cancer. But that premise lasted for about six weeks, when I began hearing from all the disease groups—heart, liver, lungs, polio, mental health, MS, diabetes, etc.—all seeking a forum for their problems.

The column has proved to be a tremendously enriching experience. I'm again in touch with remarkable people who share a common bond: coping with chronic disease and its impact on family life. My readers talk about problems, offer their own coping strategies, and continually impress me with their inventiveness and courage.

Much of this book comes from them, from the Call-PAC clients, and from the many, many others who've called and written over the years. The concerns they express, their ways of meeting powerful challenges— all are here in one form or another.

I have learned and continue to learn so much. Every time the phone rings or the mail comes I'm given a new story, a new challenge, a new opportunity.

Part Two
WHAT WE LEARNED

5
The Opposite of Fear
Is Knowledge

Geo: No one has ever been cured of cancer by ignoring it.

I discovered there are only two ways of dealing with a life-threatening illness: either you fight and give yourself a chance to live, or you surrender. I decided to fight and discovered that fear is the biggest enemy.

Fearing cancer is almost harder than having it. Fear is what makes you delay in seeking treatment. Fear is what cripples your ability to deal with it, and fear ultimately can be fatal, but cancer doesn't necessarily have to be.

Patients have questions about their disease that are not answered by their physicians, fears that are not shared with their families and not allayed by their ministers, problems that are not solved even when help is available because, too often, patients mask their true needs.

There is no magic potion that blots out these thoughts, and the going can get rough. But in order to

87

survive, you must distinguish between imaginary threats and fact. Only then will you be free to face your real challenge.

WHY DON'T WE ASK?

Not understanding their doctors and being afraid to ask them questions are the two most troublesome problems people are confronted with. In fact, these issues outrank all the other questions I've been asked over the years.

Many patients are afraid to ask their doctors important questions because they do not want to use up the doctor's valuable time. Although doctors are very busy, most want their patients to understand their conditions and the treatments they might recommend.

Here's a scenario related to me with slight variations more times than I can count. It illustrates what often goes on in a patient's mind when he sees his doctor, especially if he's meeting him for the first time.

Walter has gone to his family doctor, with whom he is comfortable, because he has abdominal pains. After his examination, Doctor X says, "Get dressed, and then we'll talk." Walter's anxiety begins to build. It must be serious, he thinks, if the doctor wants me in his office to talk about it.

Doctor X tells Walter he doesn't like what he sees, wants him to have tests performed, and refers him to a colleague whom he describes as "the best in the business." He says nothing more. Walter asks no questions but thinks, Boy, it must be serious. He says I need the best. Maybe it's cancer. Maybe I'm dying.

He leaves Doctor X's office anxious and bewildered. Ten days go by before Walter can see Doctor Y, because he's away at a medical conference. By then Walter's anxiety has heightened to the point at which he's ready to jump out of his skin.

The big day arrives. Walter approaches the door to

Doctor Y's office and sees "Oncology—General Surgery." That upsets him even more. He was hoping he had only a hernia. Inside, he gives the nurse his name, and she gives him a three-page form to fill out. The waiting room is crowded, and as Walter is trying to concentrate on his medical questionnaire several other patients are discussing their cancer surgery with each other. By now, Walter is going crazy and wants to escape.

One hour passes, then two. Finally, after another half hour goes by, the nurse calls him into an examining room, informs him the doctor will be with him shortly, hands him a paper gown, and tells him to get undressed. He wonders: His trousers? His underwear? Shoes and socks? Just what is this Doctor Y looking for anyway? Walter's anxiety has now heightened so much he looks out the window and wonders how much damage he'll sustain if he tries to jump from the sixth floor. Just then, Doctor Y walks in, cool, calm, confident, his lab coat white and crisp, his hand extended. Walter doesn't know whether to shake hands or keep his paper gown closed.

He sits on the examining table and waits, nervous and jumpy, as the doctor looks over his chart. He's worried, scared, and furious at how long he had to wait. Most of all, he's intimidated as he sits there totally undressed, covered only by a paper gown, while the guy standing above him is wearing his suit, shirt, and tie.

But Doctor Y sees a flustered and inarticulate patient who is worried about himself. He probes, pokes, and asks questions. Walter feels like a steer at an auction and wishes he could run away. But he's trapped. He knows he has pain, that something is wrong and must be corrected, but the man he trusts, old Doctor X, can't do it. He has to entrust his life to a stranger who's seen him just this one time—at his worst.

Most doctors are aware of their patient's discomfort in this situation and try to put him at ease. Nevertheless, many patients complain that some doctors do nothing to relieve their distress and that others are oblivious to it.

The overwhelming majority of doctors are highly competent, honorable, and committed to giving the best care they possibly can. Perhaps the most important element in ensuring that care is the first encounter between doctor and patient.

Walter's case pointed out how unsatisfying that first encounter can be. But everyone shared the blame—Doctor X, who didn't explain anything; Doctor Y, who intimidated Walter; and Walter, for not asking questions.

Doctors often walk into an examining room not knowing what they'll run into. The patient might be cranky or uncooperative. He may resist treatment; worst yet, he may not be treatable, and the doctor will have to pass along the unwanted news. Sometimes the doctor has to make an instant decision on how much he thinks the patient wants to hear. If he says more than the patient can hear or if he says it in the wrong way, he may frighten him so much he'll decline or delay treatment, and that may cost the patient his life.

The doctor's job is to make a diagnosis and recommend treatment. If a patient refuses to accept his judgment, the doctor can point out the risks, but the final decision is the patient's.

That doesn't mean the doctor will be personally unaffected. His concern for the person may be no less than his concern for the patient.

Our good friend, Tass Nassos, is an outstanding surgeon who receives many cancer referrals but is also introduced to patients in the emergency room after they've had serious accidents—not the easiest of circumstances. The patients have varying degrees of injuries, are anxious and frightened. If family members are there, they're often in a state of panic themselves.

While cancer is a life-threatening disease, in the emergency rooms he's often confronted with life and death decisions. Both situations are very stressful.

Tass says doctors have to gain the patients' trust. He never lies to them or bluffs them or tries to do anything that will abrogate that trust. "Abrogating that trust," he says, "means things never will be right in the doctor-patient relationship."

In fact, he says, he sometimes allows an hour or more, if necessary, until he's comfortable that he's answered all the questions the patient or family might have.

GETTING THE ANSWERS

Bud: It is very important for the patient to take the lead in keeping the lines of communication open. The best way to communicate with your doctor is to ask your questions and be sure you understand the answers.

To ask the most effective questions, you need a general understanding of your illness. When the doctor first gives you your diagnosis, ask him to refer you to some pamphlets that will give you more general information.

Before your next appointment, write down your questions and take them with you. If you think you're going to need extra time, try to inform the office staff well in advance so that they can schedule your appointment accordingly. If possible, take a family member along. When you're under stress, it's very difficult to remember what was said. An extra pair of ears can assist recall and spare repetition. Whenever Geo's doctor presented a treatment plan, she always asked, "Would you recommend this to your wife [husband/child]? Faced with a similar choice, what would you do? Why?"

If you ask similar questions, you'll find the answers very useful.

Remember these things about a doctor-patient relationship. Recognize that every patient is vying for the doctor's immediate and undivided attention, and obviously everyone can't possibly have it.

Doctors deal with hundreds of patients and there are countless other stressful demands on their time. You certainly can't expect them to adapt their personalities and approach to accommodate every patient. Nor can you expect them to guess your level of need for information. Make your wishes clear.

Some doctors, just like other people, do not feel comfortable with patients or families facing what might be a life-threatening illness. They may appear to lack understanding and empathy, although they might only be trying to protect their patients from information that may upset them. The doctors in these situations may not volunteer detailed information about the illness unless the patients confront them. You may want to reassure your doctor that knowing the information, whether good or bad, is important to you and that you are prepared to hear the truth.

On the other hand, if you do not want a lot of information, say so. And tell your doctor whom (spouse, family member, important other) you designate as the appropriate person to receive reports.

If you trust your doctor and want to continue as his or her patient, do whatever you can to ensure that your visit is productive and satisfying.

WHEN COMMUNICATION GOES AWRY

Geo: It is not always apparent to the doctor that a patient does not understand something, however. In fact, I recall on one occasion a doctor told me by phone that my x-rays revealed "an absence of mammary tissue." That bewildered me because he spoke rapidly and I could hardly absorb everything he was saying.

I thought he said "abscess" instead of "absence," and

when I asked him, he responded with annoyance and said, "For God's sake, you know you've had both breasts removed. What's your problem?" But I'd never heard that term used to describe bilateral mastectomies, and I didn't grasp it right away.

Since doctors cannot anticipate our every concern and fear, we must make it easier for them to explain to us. They are dealing with so many patients, each with a different personality and with a different ability to cope.

Some patients and their families want and need to know as much as they possibly can. Others bury their heads and feel that if there was anything crucially important the doctor would have told them. Doctors aren't mind readers. Often they explain only what they think is necessary and expect the patient to ask for additional information. But when we mishear, we don't always know it.

Once I overheard a conversation in a surgical lounge where a family spoke with the doctor who had just performed a mastectomy on their loved one. He said, "There was no involvement in the nodes," meaning the cancer had not spread to the surrounding lymph nodes, which is actually very good news.

But the family, numbed by shock, asked the doctor no further questions. Later, I heard them talking with each other about how bad it must be if the doctor had checked to see if it had spread as far as the nose! They didn't know that the lymph system runs throughout the body; that the doctor was referring to lymph nodes close to the breast; that, in fact, he was trying to reassure them. Not understanding caused unnecessary turmoil, pain, and anxiety.

Even when we do understand, mistakes happen. When I developed meningitis after my brain surgery, I was taken to the nuclear medicine department for a check of the shunt that had been implanted. A technician gave me a cup of barium to swallow. "Not this time," I said, knowing I was there for a brain scan, not a gastrointestinal series. But he insisted, saying my doctors wanted to check my internal organs to see how far the cancer had spread.

I was shocked. I started to scream. I was filled with rage, thinking that everyone important to me—my husband, my doctors, my friends—had betrayed me by concealing the truth about my condition.

My husband never had lied to me, and my doctors always had given me the facts. But suddenly I felt that everyone had lied, that the brain cyst had been malignant, that everyone was being nice to me because I did not have long to live.

I had a right to know if I was dying, I thought, especially after the long fight I had waged against my illness.

After what seemed like an eternity, another technician ran out to tell me there had been a computer error, that the GI series was scheduled for another patient. I was not scheduled for that test; there had been no spread of cancer; the cyst was, indeed, benign; no one had lied to me.

Lousy computers! I was relieved, but I'll never forget the forty minutes I spent in that lab that day. The feeling of total betrayal enraged and frightened me. Had my cousin, Joanne, not been there with me, I'd have gone crazy.

It was an error, but it also was a failure of communication. Had I not protested, I probably would have undergone the test, suffered more, and, even though the tests would have come back negative, probably never trusted anyone again.

You have to know what's being done to you, where you're being taken, what tests are being performed. Ask and make sure you get answers. And if you see a mistake has been made, don't be afraid to put everyone straight. Mistakes aren't made on purpose, but you

won't know if there has been one if you don't know
what's supposed to happen.

TREATMENT DECISIONS

Every treatment has benefits and risks. When your
doctor recommends a control program, he should outline it. Sometimes the diagnosis, coupled with a flood of
information about treatment options, leaves you too
exhausted to cope, much less make instant choices.

Fortunately, you probably won't have to decide everything right away. Ask if you can take a day or two (a
week?) to digest the information and evaluate the suggestions.

Is There a "Best" Treatment?

The answer to this question depends upon your particular diagnosis: the primary site (where the cancer
first developed), cell type, how far the cancer has
spread to other parts of the body, and your general
physical condition.

The National Cancer Institute maintains a computer
network for physicians (PDQ; see One Thing More . . .)
that includes treatment-of-choice statements for certain sites. These are based on the collective experience
of cancer specialists throughout the United States. But
even treatment-of-choice statements allow for variables
according to individual circumstances. Your "best
treatment" involves the accumulated knowledge about
cancer control applied to your specific needs. This is
what you have hired a physician to do.

Your Doctor

In the best of circumstances, your doctor has both an
appropriate medical background and good communication skills. He or she explains clearly what management

choices best fit your particular case—why the doctor is proposing a certain course of treatment. As we have said before, you have a responsibility here, too: if you don't understand, *ask*.

Who the doctor is also varies according to circumstance. If your family physician plans to treat the case, find out how much experience he or she has had with your diagnosis. Is the doctor following a plan designed by a specialist (not uncommon in areas far from treatment centers)? If the doctor refers you to other physicians, it is appropriate to ask in what subspecialty the doctors are board-certified.

How many physicians will be involved? Who is in charge of what? Sometimes you see physicians from several subspecialties and find yourself wondering, "Who is my doctor? Whom do I ask about what?" You will avoid a lot of confusion and frustration if you know the answers to these questions.

The Hospital

For this discussion, we'll consider hospitals in three somewhat oversimplified groups: community hospitals, comprehensive cancer centers, and cancer hospitals.

Community Hospitals

Your local hospital is certainly handy—but does it have the resources to meet your needs? According to the American College of Surgeons, a community hospital cancer treatment program should have the medical staff and equipment necessary to treat cancer, an active tumor registry to keep track of all patients and their treatment results, an ongoing education program for the medical staff, and regular tumor board meetings.

The college reviews hospital cancer programs throughout the country, so it's helpful to ask whether the Joint Commission on Cancer of the American College of Surgeons has awarded "full approval" to your hospital's cancer program. If not, why not?

Comprehensive Cancer Centers

Some institutions, usually teaching hospitals associated with a medical school, carry the designation Comprehensive Cancer Center, which they received from the National Cancer Institute. Comprehensive Cancer Centers often organize clinical trials, train physicians in cancer subspecialties, and offer consultation and direction to other institutions in their area.

It is not always necessary for you to go to such a center, since in many cases the treatment offered at your community hospital is the same. However, if you have a relatively rare type of cancer, these centers are likely to have more experience with its management.

Cancer Hospitals

There are two famous hospitals in the United States, Memorial Sloan-Kettering in New York City, and M.D. Anderson in Houston, Texas, that admit only cancer patients. They have become known as "cancer hospitals." Like the comprehensive cancer centers, these hospitals can take advantage of their large number of patients to conduct clinical trials; however, in many cases the treatment is no different from what you would receive nearer your home.

Your doctor can contact the appropriate physicians at either hospital, quickly outline your case, and discover whether there are any treatment protocols which are not available locally, that could apply beneficially to you.

SECOND OPINIONS

Bud: It's not always necessary to get a second opinion, and deciding when to do so is not always easy, but there

are certain things that can point you in the right direction.

If you're not happy with your doctor's methods,
manner, or reputation and you have little confidence in
him or her, it's obvious you should find someone else.
And, if you're growing weaker even though your doctor
says there's nothing seriously wrong with you, that's
another clue.

Many years ago, before I knew anything about
cancer, my father was being treated with sulfa drugs
because his doctor, an old family friend, didn't want to
tell him or us he had metastatic prostate cancer. As he
became weaker and weaker, it became obvious he was
not suffering from a cold, and I asked the doctor what
was happening. It was then he leveled with me and said
my father's illness was terminal. Although I was young
and uninformed, I still was able to insist that he refer us
to someone who might help him, and he did. My father
received treatment that gave him a few more years of
rather robust life.

More commonly, patients seek a second opinion because they have a serious illness and are uncertain or
uncomfortable about their physician's recommendation. Since cancer is by definition a serious disease, a
second opinion is appropriate—especially if an unusual
or highly intrusive form of treatment is involved.

One man called Geo after he left his doctor's office
devastated because he had been told to check into the
hospital for a colostomy. When he tried to ask questions, the doctor said, "Don't worry about a thing. I'll
take care of all the arrangements. Your job is to get
yourself to the hospital on Sunday at three o'clock."

When the man went home and told his wife everything, she became frightened and upset, too. She was
frightened by the prospect of cancer and a colostomy
and upset that her husband had been left so ill informed
about important decisions concerning his life.

The wife had many valid questions, the most important being, How did the doctor determine that her husband needed the colostomy? He had gone in to be examined because of a change in bowel habits. Second, she wanted to know who would be doing the surgery, since her husband's doctor was an internist.

She set the wheels in motion and, within three days, had arranged for a complete evaluation with a cancer surgeon elsewhere who determined that her husband did not need surgery at all.

Her actions spared her husband needless pain, surgery, and worry.

If you want a second opinion, you may (1) ask your family physician to suggest a specialist, (2) contact the American Cancer Society or the National Cancer Institute for information about cancer hospitals and community cancer programs, or (3) if you have a particular hospital in mind, call and ask for the chairman of the Cancer Committee, who will refer you to the right specialist.

Remember that a second opinion will have meaning only if it is based on the same medical information as the first—your history, test results, and the records of treatments given, if any. Thus, arrangements must include the collection of your medical records.

There are no firm rules for getting a second opinion. Many people have complete confidence in one doctor, remain under his or her care for the entire course of the disease, and receive excellent care. Others may want verification of the diagnosis or a proposed course of treatment. The decision is yours.

MEDICAL RECORDS

Geo: The legal rights of patients vary according to state laws. In some states, access to technical information in medical records is not allowed, while others require only that general information be given to patients. Sometimes states allow doctors to refuse access to records if they feel that this information would be "harmful" to the patient. Still other states have laws assuring the right to records in almost all cases.

But many patients have a strong interest in the information in their records, so there's been a trend toward increasing patient access to them—particularly now that most insurance companies request second opinions before they will pay for procedures and operations.

If you would like to obtain copies of your medical records, talk to your doctor first. If you're seeking them for a second opinion at another facility, the doctor or hospital may agree to make them available but may insist that they be mailed directly to the consulting physician. Others may give the records directly to the patient. In either case it is appropriate to get an introductory cover letter from the referring physician.

Although they shouldn't, some physicians do resent a patient's getting a second opinion. They feel that the patient is questioning their competence and diagnosis. These doctors might feel threatened because there is so much uncertainty regarding the disease and the various modes of treatment that no one really can offer a guarantee.

The situation can be uncomfortable, particularly if the consulting physician agrees with the diagnosis and treatment and you choose to return to your original doctor. This causes the doctor-patient relationship to erode somewhat, and you might feel intimidated. But remember, the second opinion sometimes means the difference between life and death. Remember, too, that if your physician is a specialist, he or she may frequently be asked to give a second opinion and will therefore understand your request.

I recently went through the experience of compiling many years of medical records pertaining to my breast cancer and brain surgery to send to a top research facility in San Francisco for an evaluation. In my instance, it meant getting medical records from four hospitals and eight doctors. What makes my case perplexing is that the cyst on the brain was benign, despite the fact that the breast cancer had spread to my lymph nodes.

Even though my cancer surgeon and neurosurgeon are very highly regarded and extremely competent, I felt it was crucial to pursue every possible avenue available to me. This pursuit has been one of the reasons I've survived so long and so well.

The California evaluation determined that nothing could or should be done. Since they agreed with my present physicians that the condition is untreatable and inoperable, I'll continue to be under their care because I trust them.

UNPROVEN CANCER REMEDIES

Bud: Sometimes, when traditional procedures appear unable to control the disease, the patient and family begin to consider unproven remedies. Enormous pressure is exerted by well-meaning friends and colleagues to leave no stone unturned in the quest for survival. The distraught patient receives a barrage of unsolicited information when he or she is most vulnerable and the patient, together with family, has difficulty evaluating what is valid. Frequently, other patients push these methods through an underground that exists.

These "treatments" include special diets, secret herbal teas, powerful vitamins, laetrile, psychosurgery, urine extract tablets, meditation, and the laying on of hands. The tabloids usually herald these so-called breakthroughs, as they did when the actor Steve McQueen went to Mexico after he discontinued his chemotherapy treatments. They fail to mention the thousands who have died from these so-called cures, however.

Chronic disorders, like arthritis, cancer, and Alzheimer's disease, are popular targets. How can you evaluate claims for cures? Ask these questions:

1. Does the claimant offer personal testimonials, rather than controlled, repeatable studies to document results?
2. Does the claimant request payment in advance? Has your insurance company refused to cover costs?
3. Does the claimant refuse to reveal the "secret" of the treatment and describe the "medical establishment" as an enemy? (Reputable physicians and institutions share their work; they don't hide it.)
4. Does the drug (or treatment, or substance, or diet) supposedly have properties that will cure more than one disease?
5. Are claims for the product printed by an organization that will make money from its sale?

If the answer to any one of these questions is "yes," beware.

Sometimes a cultlike following develops for a specific "cure." Pressure is not necessarily felt by the medical professionals because patients are reluctant to inform their doctors about their interest in exploring alternate therapies. But pressure and emotional turmoil cause patients to seriously consider pursuing these remedies.

It is not only the poor and less knowledgeable who consider these alternatives. Wealthy, well-educated, and sophisticated people do also.

Geo was offered many "cures" when she first became ill and opted for conventional treatment. Then, when new cancers developed and she became more visible through her lecturing and television appearances, the pressure from some groups was relentless. They hounded us day and night with phone calls and mysterious messages that had a way of popping up at our home and even in our grocery bags. It was rough riding this out.

But we knew that avoiding standard treatments would be running away and that Geo's only hope lay in confronting her cancer and doing what needed to be done to control it.

If there was one thing we didn't want, it was to be victimized twice—once by the disease—and again by an alleged cure.

HEALTH INSURANCE

Most of us tend to take our health insurance for granted. Our experience says that's a mistake. Next to serious illness itself, medical bills are the greatest source of family stress. If your coverage is inadequate, you need to know early on so that you can take steps to get help.

If you are fortunate enough to have good coverage, you must try to preserve it—your situation may make it impossible to change jobs.

Sometimes it may make getting a job impossible in the first place or accepting one beneath your level of training or competence.

Ron was twenty-one when he learned he had testicular cancer. Because he was a college student he was covered by his father's insurance plan. He underwent surgery and radiation and, after a recurrence, twelve months of grueling chemotherapy. He was optimistic, looking forward to complete recovery, never even dreaming that his illness would affect his job opportunities when he received his degree a year later.

He breezed through job interviews, his prospective employers obviously impressed and pleased until the very end when they asked about his health. When he told them that he had had cancer, their tone changed. All interviews, Ron said, ended abruptly.

"We'll be in touch," he was told, but no one ever got back to him. Eventually, after much searching and much more disappointment, Ron did find a job. It wasn't one he was trained for, or one that earned him a

living wage, but one which did, at least, provide medical insurance for everything except his preexisting
condition.

Six years later, Ron's cancer has not reappeared, he
has not missed a single day of work, but he has still
been unable to find a job more suited to his abilities.

As countless families have told us, coping with both
the illness and its financial consequences constitutes a
terrific strain. Nevertheless, learn exactly where you
stand so that any decisions you make will be informed
ones and problems will not surface without warning.

Be sure you understand completely what is and is not
going to be paid for by your insurance company.

If it appears your personal costs will be more than
you can afford, make an appointment with the hospital
medical social worker, who can advise you about support from government and community resources.

Save every bill, every receipt, *every* piece of paper
you receive related to medical costs. Make copies of
everything you file with an insurance claim. Should a
claim be rejected, you may wish to refile or appeal.
Some expenses not covered by insurance may be tax-
deductible.

6
Coping with Treatment

GET INVOLVED AND KEEP TRACK

Geo: A cancer diagnosis is shocking; dealing with its treatment is draining. But most people have within them the resources to cope—though at first they may not know it.

Successful coping, we've learned, occurs when people get involved and when they ask themselves not "How can I stand this?" but "What can I do about it?"

Being involved in your care means talking directly with your doctor, learning what he or she is planning to do and why. It means making your own arrangements for treatments and return visits and keeping a calendar.

Find a good calendar that has plenty of space for all your appointments—personal and medical. Encourage everyone in the house to add information and consult it regularly before making plans.

If you have more medications than you can easily

keep track of, make a daily chart for each drug, its dose, and the time you have to take it. Then, as you take the medicine, check it off on the chart.

When your doctor says he or she expects test results to arrive before your next appointment, mark the due date on your calendar and call to see if the x-ray or other results have in fact arrived. If you are scheduled to visit another facility for consultation and/or treatment, ask to take your medical file with you.

And if you arrive at a laboratory or diagnostic x-ray or other testing facility, and the technician begins a procedure you did not expect, *speak up*. Ask questions. Don't assume anything.

I have a severe allergy to iodine that is injected for the kidney intravenous pyelogram (IVP) and for some scans, but it has been routinely overlooked or ignored even though it has been emblazoned on my charts. On five separate occasions clinicians were ready to inject me with iodine, even after I had made myself sound like a broken record telling them about my allergy to it.

I found it was easier to let them schedule the tests and then tell the technicians I was allergic to fish and iodine. "So what?" they asked. "So, I might die during the test," I'd reply. The procedure would be scrubbed hastily, and I'd be returned to my room. The last time it occurred to me that if I were unconscious and the technician didn't bother to check my chart, I would be in serious trouble. "Please double-check," I told my nurses. "If you can't ask me, ask my husband."

It's also wise to keep a diary of your feelings. If, during treatment, you've had twenty-five bad days and only five good ones, you'll get a psychological lift when you've reached the point where you've had only five bad ones and twenty-five good ones. Paying attention to your symptoms and your psyche helps the healing process. You'll feel better as you monitor your stress, fear, and anxiety and log your improvement.

I began my radiation therapy during the last week of October 1968, and it continued through Thanksgiving and the Christmas holidays. By Easter of 1969, I finally had begun to rebound. I knew it was futile to complain chronically even though I felt miserable and had few tolerable days, but because I also knew what to expect I did not become discouraged by a lack of visible progress. I couldn't rush things along, so all I could do was to hang in there and take it day by day. I asked questions; I tried to do small things that would make the dreary days less dreary. I kept my diary, and little by little I began to see I was having fewer side effects and more and more good days.

An important thing that healthy people should understand is that chemotherapy and radiation treatments are not therapy in the sense that whirlpool and massage are, where the more you get, the better you feel. They definitely are not a treat. Their effect is cumulative, and the more you get the more you're wiped out.

Being in touch with your symptoms and your psyche enables you to cope more effectively. It helps clear your mind of uncertainty and trivia that might weigh you down. For example, if you don't identify your feelings clearly—and their sources—during a specific procedure, you might panic if it has to be repeated. If a test was "awful," what made it so? Was the procedure painful? Or was your anxiety too great? Were you worrying about something else that day?

When a test hurts, you tend to remember the discomfort only too well. Try to think of things that will help relieve your distress. Concentrate on what will calm you down. If you have kept a journal of treatment, you'll know what helps you relax.

You Are Not a Victim

Of the many battles fought around the management of cancer, none is more powerful or more often misunderstood than the issue of control.

Health professionals complain about "noncompliant"

patients. Patients complain that their doctors don't care about them or their feelings.

Everyone involved needs to remember that the patients have lost a precious commodity: control of their lives. Normal patterns of living have been sacrificed to medical appointments that are made at the convenience of the medical center. Things are done *to* the patients that are invasive and uncomfortable. They have a disease—the uncontrolled growth of cells—that reflects how their lives have been upset; its management will involve further loss of control.

Small wonder, then, that patients sometimes react by refusing treatments or missing appointments. They seem cranky and demanding about trivial issues. I'm *not* talking here about being offered a treatment option and, after discussing the risks and benefits carefully, deciding not to proceed. I *am* talking about hasty, obviously emotion-laden declarations where the patients, in effect, dig in their heels and say no.

The best way to deal with the issue of control is, of course, head-on. If patients and doctors work together to grant the patients the largest measure of control possible, the patients can function as members of the health care team—not merely as its objects.

Patients must recognize this need in themselves, so that instead of saying, "I don't care what you say, I'm not having surgery," they can say, "It's important for me to know as much as possible and to participate as much as possible in the decisions that affect my life. Let's work together on this."

Health care professionals and family members, in turn, must avoid turning patients into helpless children, making all decisions and treating the patients as incompetent. One young woman I know (caring for her father who had a brain tumor) reported the following incident: "One night Dad got up at 2:00 A.M. and went to the bathroom to shower and shave. When I tried to stop him and get him back to bed, he exclaimed, 'I don't like people telling me *when* I can do something!' On reflection, I realized he was right—what difference did it make *when* he took his shower? The tumor was stealing his life. Scheduling personal tasks was the last measure of control left to him—and I tried to take that, too!"

I am reminded of the man who called our listening service, distraught because his seventeen-year-old nephew, Ronald, was refusing a leg amputation for sarcoma. The young man had been injured during a ballgame, but the x-rays revealed a malignancy rather than a fracture.

Ronald's family pressured him into allowing the surgery to take place immediately. Not only did he refuse, he ran away for three weeks. When he returned, he informed his family that the surgery could take place on September 15, the day after his eighteenth birthday. Since he had no control over the diagnosis, he wanted to sign his own surgical release form, which he did.

In another case, Mary, a terminal patient confined to a hospital isolation ward, had an intensely personal request. She wanted to leave the hospital so she could experience sexual intercourse for the first time.

She had spent almost her entire adult life paying her parents' hospital bills. Both had died of cancer. She hadn't finished paying those bills, and now she was unable to pay her own. She had worked so hard that she never had time to date, never even had a boyfriend until now, when, at age thirty-six, she was dying.

Mary told me her friend was sincere, attentive, and loyal, loved her even if she had cancer, and visited her daily, putting on a mask, gown, and gloves and going through the necessary precautions in order to spend a few minutes with her.

Her doctors refused to release her, saying she was too ill, but Mary insisted that she spend whatever time she had left at home with her boyfriend. She had been afraid to tell them her true reason, because she didn't want anyone to think of her as "that kind of woman." Fortunately, she confided in me, and I was able to pass along her request to an understanding chaplain who arranged for her discharge. She spent the rest of her life—ten days—at home with the man she loved. Those days meant more to her than an extra few weeks of life isolated in the hospital. Finally, Mary told me, she felt she was taking charge. She had not been able to control her life; she *did* control her death.

It's your body and your treatment. You'd better become involved and start asking questions. Accept help as you need it, but don't relinquish your responsibility to yourself. Don't become an invalid for whom others assume control and make decisions.

Being in charge means more than being an informed medical consumer. It means getting second opinions. It means asking questions even if you think they're stupid or insignificant. Anything that is causing you distress deserves an answer. Don't push your questions aside; you'll find they keep resurfacing.

A twenty-six-year-old man I know, engaged to be married, undergoing treatment for testicular cancer, asked me some so-called insignificant questions he hadn't asked his physicians. What were those "insignificant" questions? "Will I become sterile from this treatment? Will they have any effect on sexual intercourse?"

Those questions were neither insignificant nor stupid. In fact, it was imperative that he and his fiancee know the answers. Since his caregivers hadn't brought up the subject, he felt his concerns were inappropriate or irrelevant, and they were anything but.

Not being a victim doesn't mean you sidestep pain or stress or loss. It *does* mean you have learned what to expect and decided how you're going to cope.

MIRROR, MIRROR

Emotional ups and downs are to be expected when one is stricken with cancer, but we usually don't know all the physical changes to anticipate.

Following brain surgery, I was placed on steroids to

reduce the inflammation of the brain. While this treatment is very effective, it does have side effects, such as a "moonface," where you're so puffed up, you don't even resemble yourself. The steroids cause your body to retain fluid, creating a weight gain.

I gained eighteen pounds, none of my clothes fit me, and I couldn't stand to look at myself in a mirror.

The hair on my head grew in thick and silky, and so did my eyelashes. It also grew where I didn't need or want it, such as on my face and arms. I became accustomed to strange expressions when people told me a "hair-raising" tale and the hair on my arms stood up two inches.

Although our bathroom had double wash basins, I didn't want to overdo the togetherness bit with my husband by shaving at the same time every morning, so I opted for wax removal treatments. When the steroids were discontinued, my hair fell out again and I lost weight.

I hadn't had problems dealing with the removal of both breasts or with the need to wear wigs, but the facial hair and moon face created a lot of conflict within me. I was amazed and overjoyed by the remarkable recovery I had made, but I was distressed with the change in my appearance.

While my side effects were temporary, many people are continuously on steroid treatment. Patients with debilitating neuromuscular diseases must not only adjust to physical pain and limitations but must also learn to live with side effects that significantly alter their body image.

Acceptance of these things is difficult at best, and mood swings are significantly attached to how you look.

A large part of the problem for the patient is that friends don't want to deal with it: they don't want to feel that their own appearance could be altered. Their refusal to accept your new look makes it even more difficult for you to cope.

For a while I thought I was probably the only one who

couldn't accept these kinds of changes or the way healthy people reacted to them. I guess because I'm so open I was able to brush aside comments friends made, comments they thought were encouraging, such as, "Don't worry so much. You look fine!" or "Big deal—so you've put on some weight," with a combination of confrontation and flippancy.

Sometimes I'd say, "It's not easy to look into a mirror and see someone you don't recognize" or "Fortunately, I'll be on this medication only for two months," etc. Other times I'd respond, "How would you feel if you lost your hair or saw your face puff up?"

They'd get the message, but I ran the risk of having them consider me hostile or cranky. I found the best way to overcome it was with a sense of humor.

After I gained twenty pounds, I'd joke that Bud liked big women and I wanted to please him. Or I'd say, "He has a fetish for bald women."

I've never considered myself a sex symbol, so I never gave any consideration to posing for *Playboy* magazine. But when I served as a consultant to the National Cancer Institute, Harvard Medical School was in the process of preparing a new medical manual. They needed photographs of a premenopausal, bilateral mastectomy patient who had undergone radiation therapy. "Imagine that," I told Bud, "your wife—a Harvard centerfold!"

Always keep in mind that if you look in the mirror and see someone you don't recognize, just close your eyes and focus on what you used to look like. The *person* that is you hasn't changed. Only your outer wrapper has changed.

ON RADIATION/CHEMOTHERAPY

When I was halfway through my radiation treatments, we were invited to a christening. Most of our friends there were thrilled to see me up and around, but I don't think they realized that I wanted to be with them so much, I didn't want to leave.

In fact, I didn't want the evening to end. Bud was concerned that I would overdo it and be too exhausted to go for my treatment the next morning. I recall that I was terrified of dying, but as long as I stayed in the company of my well friends, I didn't seem to dwell on it. I wanted that Sunday night to last forever.

I guess that was my anxiety showing and a denial that my life was being threatened. At the party I could feel my illness was all a bad dream. (Too bad it wasn't!)

One woman told me her sixty-eight-year-old mother had become depressed and withdrawn since she had begun radiation treatment. She wasn't aware that many patients under treatment are upset to some degree. While radiation may affect the emotions indirectly through fatigue or changes in hormone balance, it in itself is not a direct cause of mental distress.

Patients often report being anxious, depressed, or nervous during their radiation and chemotherapy treatments. These feelings may have a number of sources: a change in daily routines, limits on their mobility, fear of the disease, and most of all, fear of dying. These are common emotions after a diagnosis of cancer.

If this woman had discussed these things with her mother, she might have been able to ease some of her anxiety. This might have helped her mother to direct less of her much-needed energy into worrying and more into getting through her treatments.

I recall in 1968–69 when I received my radiation, no one talked about it, and I felt the same kind of worry. But because the medical profession frowned on patient-to-patient contact, we weren't allowed to talk with other patients for fear we would compare situations and symptoms. I didn't know others experienced distress, and I thought something was very wrong with me.

In addition, the staff never explained things or expressed concern about our fears and anxieties. All in
all, receiving radiation at that time was lonely, frightening, and depressing.

I remember with sadness one occasion when a man
came to pick up his elderly mother after treatment. She
was sobbing, and he asked her what was wrong. She
said she was sick and felt weak and nauseated.

He then turned to the technicians and asked them if
something had hurt or upset his mother. They replied
no, and failed to explain that the treatment itself often
causes weariness, nausea, depression. Then the son told
his mother that the doctors had said nothing was wrong
with her, so she'd better pull herself together and stop
her whimpering.

He seemed angry and annoyed with her. She slowly
arose and walked out behind her son like a rejected
puppy. I felt so sorry for her. I was fortunate that my
husband and family listened and believed me when I
told them how I felt.

Both radiation and chemotherapy are powerful weap-
ons against cancer, but they do have side effects. For
me, it was like having severe flulike symptoms that
never seemed to end. But when the treatments ended
and I began to feel better, I could look upon the radiation as a friend that had helped save my life. When no
improvement is apparent, some patients question the
need to continue treatments—like Ann, who decided to
discontinue hers. She had undergone surgery, radiation, and chemotherapy. Shortly before she called me,
her doctors had told her that additional treatments
were necessary because of a recurrence.

Ann had been under continual treatment since her
diagnosis three years before and felt she had no quality
of life—that she was merely existing from day to day.
She preferred to stay home and spend time with her
family and friends even though she knew she wasn't

going to survive for very long. Her family, unwilling to let go, tried to change her mind, which made her remaining days uncomfortable. She told me several weeks before she died that they were still nagging her about resuming the treatments. But she had made her decision.

I'll never forget Mark, who pursued his treatments as he pursued his life, with great intensity. Because it was important for him to go sailing with his friends on weekends, he rearranged his schedule. He worked for a bank, finished early on Wednesdays, had a chemotherapy treatment promptly after work, then went home "to throw up," as he described it. He felt weak and nauseated on Thursdays, but it didn't keep him from going to work. By Friday, he had recovered and was able to enjoy his weekend. Having plans gave him the incentive to endure his treatment.

Mary, on the other hand, told me that all she did from week to week was stay home and be miserable. I asked her to try several things. Since she always had anxiety before her treatments, I told her to find something she enjoyed doing the night before, such as going to the movies, going out with her friends, or playing bingo. Since she felt too weak to eat after her treatment, I suggested that she go for lunch before her treatment. She tried these suggestions and called me back.

She and her husband agreed to go to a movie, preferably a comedy, every Tuesday night, and she had lunch with her sister, who drove her to the treatment. It picked up her spirits enough that she said it made a world of difference for her emotionally.

OVERCOMING PAIN

Pain comes in varying degrees, ranging from bearable and manageable to excruciating, unrelenting, and unbearable. Some days I found it debilitating and exhausting; but sometimes, while undergoing certain procedures that I fully expected to hurt, I was surprised by the pain that wasn't there.

Postsurgical pain is often the most severe, but it can be controlled with medication. Unfortunately, many patients don't know whether their doctor has left a "medication on demand" order. And right after an operation, you are likely to be too groggy and confused to know if it's time for a shot. Therefore, *always* report pain at once; the nurses may simply be waiting to hear from you.

Most pain, whether acute or chronic, can be managed. Cancer patients and many who suffer from other illnesses sometimes have such excruciating and continual pain that it becomes a psychic companion. When medication no longer is helpful, they search for new ways to manage it. Some turn to biofeedback; others learn relaxation techniques and stress management, still others undergo specialized surgery to reduce theirs.

Pain and anxiety are difficult to separate, since one tends to heighten the other. Worries can make pain seem more severe. And pain often causes worry—about its control or what it might be indicating. Thus most effective pain control programs address both pain and stress.

Somewhere along the way you may develop a tolerance for pain. I found over the years that, since I was in constant pain, a trip to the dentist was a lark, even for root canal work. Since I'm allergic to most pain medications, I tell myself I have no choice but to grit my teeth, hold on tight, and bear it.

Some days I'm in terrible pain, but I refuse to stay in bed because I've found being busy helps me focus on what I'm doing and not on my pain. It's worked for me.

To explore what will work for you, talk with your physician and/or the American Cancer Society and the National Cancer Institute (see One Thing More . . .).

Both organizations offer excellent materials on pain management and can refer you to pain control clinics.

STRESS

The emotional stress of living with cancer can cloud your thinking and push you into decisions that will make things worse than they already are.

A young father who learned his terminally ill wife would be allowed to leave the hospital to be with him and their five children for the Christmas holidays prepared to put their home up for sale because she was too ill to go upstairs to their bedroom.

He was so overwhelmed by his problems he failed to see there was a much simpler solution. He could get a hospital bed and other equipment free of charge from the American Cancer Society and put it on the first floor, where his wife could be in the center of the family's activities.

A few years ago a lot of attention was focused on a newly developed scale that measured stress levels. Major life events were rated, and the death of a loved one and the onset of a serious illness were at the top.

Virtually no one can avoid the frustrating, irritating, maddening, never-ending hassles that occur almost every day, but researchers are finding that how well we cope with daily hassles is an indicator of how well we would be able to cope with genuine crises.

Some people deal with each crisis as it arises and then move on with their lives. But some people suffer so much stress, it debilitates them physically and emotionally.

The symptoms include irritability, sleeplessness, headaches, fatigue, loss of appetite or overeating, panic attacks, ulcers, depression, and the inability to make decisions.

It is important to recognize these harmful symptoms and try to alleviate them.

- Deal with one problem at a time, one day at a time.
- Recognize the crucial difference between a situation that can be changed and one that simply must be accepted.
- Talk your problems over with someone before they overwhelm you.
- Find an outlet before the stress destroys you.
- Keep your expectations reasonable, both for yourself and for those around you.
- Learn to recognize your own responses to stress, such as a pounding heart, severe headaches, or trembling hands.
- Learn to use relaxation techniques regularly.
- Take time for yourself to play and relax.
- Set limits, both at home and at work. Practice saying no.
- Try to change your attitude, worry less.
- Above all, don't lose your sense of humor.

Bud: Some people deal with the stress brought on by illness much better than others, but stress piled upon other stress challenges even those who are by nature cheerful, confident, and optimistic.

Do you ever wonder why a superb hitter may strike out four times in a game or why a master of words might suddenly become tongue-tied? Could it have something to do with a problem at home?

No one who watched the 1988 Winter Olympics at Calgary will forget the heartbreak of Dan Jansen, the world champion sprint skater who was favored to win gold medals in the five-hundred- and one-thousand-meter races. Jansen's twenty-eight-year old sister died of leukemia the same day he was to skate his first race. Having dedicated his Olympic performances to her, he stayed on to compete but fell in the first race, was unable to finish, and lost his chance for a medal.

Four days later, in his second race, he fell again.

Dan Jansen is a superb athlete, the best in the world in his event, tested time and again under the pressures of international competition, a skater who never falls, but who did so in successive events.

It was the most important race of his life, and he could not complete it.

Stress is universal!

Nancy Reagan's mastectomy was performed on October 17, 1987. Fortunately, her tumor was noninvasive, and her prognosis was good. That had to be a giant relief to the president, as it would have been to any other husband. Having waited out that kind of surgery on my wife, I could not help wondering what was going through the president's mind. *Newsweek* magazine reported that members of the White House staff said, "Mrs. Reagan's condition weighed heavily on the president's mind before her surgery," and one insider warned that his performance in office might suffer if his wife were in poor health. It went on to say that a long illness would have a tremendous effect on the president's ability to function. He wouldn't care about anything else, and he'd "just vegetate . . . that's how much she means to him." That comes as no surprise to me. I felt the same way.

But that wasn't the only crisis the president had to face that week. In the two days preceding the first lady's surgery, two ships—one an American-owned tanker, the other a Kuwaiti tanker showing the American flag—were hit by Iranian missiles in the Persian Gulf. Two days after her surgery, on October 19, the stock market crashed, falling 508 points, the worst plunge in history. Meanwhile, the president's battle to win confirmation of Judge Robert Bork to the Supreme Court was on its way to overwhelming defeat.

Now, that's stress!

RECURRENCE

Geo: There is a tremendous feeling of relief when a patient recovers from surgery or completes other treatment because he or she finally can move away from a hospital environment. The patient is happy to have survived and now can focus on the future but still has some degree of fear and anxiety because of the possibility the disease will recur.

Some patients remain disease-free for many years, but they are understandably nervous during their regular checkups, concerned that their doctors will find "something." They find it difficult to have a "normal" illness. Every cold, every ache, every strange sensation can be magnified into a potential threat.

A recurrence can cause more acute emotional distress than a patient had at the original diagnosis, surgery, radiation, or chemotherapy. It's a terrible letdown to learn one has to do it all over again. The patient's family is also distressed. They've resumed their lifestyle, gone back to work, tried to pick up where they left off—only to have their lives interrupted again. Their fear that the patient might die is rekindled; they may become despondent and not be as supportive as they were the first time around.

Since the original treatment was painful or caused severe side effects, the patient may be reluctant or unwilling to repeat it. When I underwent surgery for my recurrence, some people said to me, "You've already been through it; it shouldn't be so bad this time." Some things may be easier the second time, but not cancer, not a recurrence.

When my friend Joan had a recurrence, she was devastated. She had pushed herself to recover quickly from her initial surgery and follow-up treatment, maintained excellent health habits, resumed her housekeeping chores, took care of her husband and son, was active in her temple, became a full-time volunteer in the American Cancer Society's Reach to Recovery program and with Call-PAC. She was a devout person and thought she had been "good." Now she felt her reward for all of this was a recurrence, and she was angry.

Joan used her anger to energize her efforts. She

reached out for support—to her family, her fellow volunteers, to the hospital pastoral counselor, to support groups—spending as much time as possible with other patients who'd had recurrences and expressed their feelings openly.

She found that her feelings of helplessness and anger were not unusual and got reassurance that she was *not* a failure. Her first illness had nothing to do with her actions; neither did the second. Her second course of treatment was rougher and went on longer than the first. But her determination—and the encouragement of others—helped her cope.

For Joan, and for many others, the discovery of recurrent disease can be shattering, no matter how prepared you think you are. Bud and I worried about cancer in my remaining breast and deliberately set out to prove or disprove it. Nonetheless, the positive pathology report was a blow.

If that happens to you, remember that while your treatment may be rougher the second time around, you've already tested your coping strengths once, and you know they work. You learned how to deal with pain, with nausea, with weariness—and you can do it again.

You also know the blessing of restored health—you can imagine being well. The treatment, however difficult, is only the means; look forward to your goal.

7
"Bad" Feelings/ "Good" Feelings

Geo: Feelings aren't good or bad; they're just feelings. You can't ignore them or simply wish them away, but they can't control what you do if you don't let them.

It's scary when someone in the family has cancer. A strange sense of confusion and loneliness afflicts every member of the family, each of whom sort of drifts off into his own little compartment, unable or unwilling, perhaps, to understand or talk about what he feels.

You must talk about your feelings, but first you have to admit you have them. Admit it to yourself, admit it to others. It may not be easy and you may think that keeping to yourself is the best way to handle the situation, but you may be surprised by how much better you feel after you've gotten them off your chest. Find someone willing to listen—good friend, pastor, or health professional.

I've talked with hundreds of patients who believed that some of the "negative" feelings they experienced were something to be ashamed of. "I can tell you, Geor-

123

gia," they'd confess, "but my family wouldn't understand."

What worried them? Most commonly, they mentioned depression, anger, and grief.

DEPRESSION

Depression is an inevitable consequence of illness. Everybody gets depressed. And everybody remembers the old saying "Laugh, and the world laughs with you; weep, and you weep alone." What they may conclude from that hackneyed phrase is that, when you're depressed you should withdraw from the world, from your friends, and tough it out alone. Wrong!

Depression (and I mean here the mild sort, not the type that requires professional intervention) is a normal consequence of being ill. You're sick; the treatments may make you sicker. You're tired. You're trying to cope with a rough situation. You wonder whether you have a future and, if you do, what it will be like. You may feel like being alone.

Be alone—but don't stay that way. The worst aspect of depression is its insidious power to make you believe that the depression itself cannot be lifted. But it can! You may *feel* depressed, but you don't have to act that way.

It's important to recognize the feeling. Share your thoughts with someone you trust who can empathize with you or understand how you feel and, at the same time, help you think of pleasant things to do.

One family I know, although saddened and stressed, opened a gathering with Champagne. "We wanted to focus on what we have to celebrate," they said, "on our joy in each other, on the good times we had, and on the good times we'll have again."

A young man with Hodgkin's disease told me he went to the movies—comedies—after treatment that left him exhausted. The comedies gave him relief when he felt particularly overwhelmed.

Plagued by thoughts that her cervical cancer would prevent a return to a normal social life, a young single woman found that she could combat her depression best by first "embracing" it. Alone in her apartment, she would weep profusely, releasing her sense of paralysis. Then she'd call a friend and say, "Let's go out. I've got to do something."

When we trained recovered cancer patients for the Call-PAC listening service, one of the chaplains asked about depression, and everyone laughed. Why? First, it was a laugh of recognition: they all knew how it felt to be down. Second, it was a laugh of survival: they kept on going and made it.

ANGER

Suppressed anger can have a debilitating effect on a patient's emotional well-being. I remember several occasions when one of my doctors did not respond to my fears and concerns. He intimidated and admonished me with every question I tried to raise. I'd leave his office very depressed and usually in tears.

But instead of telling him or writing him a letter about how I felt, I allowed it to tear at me, and it constantly caused me distress that I now know was physically and emotionally destructive. I went from month to month reliving what he said, what I should have said, and what I planned to say at the next appointment. I finally blew up (five years later), and now our relationship is one of mutual respect. In fact, I really like him, value his judgment, and talk with him freely now.

When something similar happened after my brain surgery, I was so troubled I couldn't sleep because I didn't express my anger when it surfaced. I read somewhere that Abraham Lincoln would sometimes respond to his critics and others who angered him by writing them nasty letters, then throwing them away when they were finished. Writing them got his feelings off his chest and allowed him to avoid confrontations that might have made the situation worse. So I wrote a long letter to my doctors about everything that annoyed me. I wrote and wrote, and several hours later I felt such a catharsis that I didn't need to send it!

Another member of an elite group of health professionals has responded to my fears and concerns by admonishing me and telling me that I was demanding, pushy, intrusive, and aggressive. And for this demoralizing litany, I received a bill . . . and all the questions I urgently needed answers to were placed on hold until my next appointment, four months away. Past experiences lead me to presume the same thing will happen then, also.

Now, if my prominent doctors were using these descriptive terms because I was seeking miracle cosmetic surgery to become the world's most beautiful woman, I'd think, perhaps, they were justified.

But I've been dealing with a maze of illnesses and complications that began at birth and ended with brain surgery and a shunt implant last year, followed by an excruciatingly painful bout with meningitis. And what I've needed from these physicians to whom I've entrusted my life is to level with me and treat me like the intelligent, rational, caring human being I feel I am.

I am not hostile, angry, or vengeful, and I don't want pity. Neither have I cried wolf. To the contrary, I feel great and certainly look good considering I have never had any reconstructive patchwork done.

But if I hadn't been demanding, pushy, intrusive, and aggressive on far too many occasions, I wouldn't be alive today. I was admonished when I suspected that the lump in my right breast was different from the other four that resulted in surgery for fibrocystic disease. But it *was* different, and the cancer had spread to the surrounding lymph nodes before they removed the breast. Then, following all the radiation treatments, I was told there was nothing more that could be done, but Bud and I kept searching until we learned that an oophorectomy and hysterectomy in young, pre-menopausal women might retard the spread of cancer. So, after more recurrences, those procedures were performed, too.

I was prepped for the wrong surgery in two first-rate hospitals and struggled hard to fight off the sedation to prevent the surgery from taking place while the surgical team pronounced me obstinate. The fact that I have a terrible allergy to adhesive tape used after surgery has been boldly written all over my charts and wrist identification and was totally ignored on three occasions.

My allergy to the iodine injected prior to scans has repeatedly been ignored, and technicians have asked me, "So what?" Well, I might die during the procedure, that's what! And the procedures would be hastily canceled.

Despite a stuttering that I'd developed, dizziness, driving my car off the road four times, seizures and stumbling, dropping glasses and food, difficulty in holding a pen, and falling out of bed, my complaints about these difficulties were brushed aside with the admonishment to "quit looking for problems . . . and don't worry about the cancer." Why shouldn't I? I know it can spread to the brain, and since I didn't have all these problems before, it was logical to presume there was something wrong now. Following the MRI scan that showed a massive cyst affixed to my brain and the determination that I had to have brain surgery, the doctors came right in and dumped it on me. They didn't call my husband first. There was no preparation . . . no gentle words, no hand-holding. Just straight out.

I was not only terrified but had to work out a way to break it to my loving husband, who has already logged more waiting time and anguish than anyone should ever have to experience in a

lifetime. Then I had to tell the kids, who have
known me almost all of their lives as being sick;
then our widowed mothers, sisters, priests, and
friends. As usual, everyone conveyed his initial
astonishment and fear to me. After all, I was the
one telling them what was to happen. I'd find myself time and time again, surgery after surgery,
having to suppress and work through my own fears
and conflict in some sort of hiding place while I
helped everyone else handle their worry about me.

My "hiding place" is a church or hospital chapel,
and it's the only place where I can really let go. In
fact, when I first became ill, I made an arrangement with God that, in return for the gift of life, I
would be a source of inspiration to all the sick and
sorrowing people who approached me for help. I've
kept my part of the bargain, and so has God.

That's what our relationship is all about. He
talks, I listen, I ask, He listens . . . and I guess that's
a lot more than my doctors do.

When I developed meningitis, the nurses were
great when I was cheerful and cooperative. But
this all changed when I became frustrated and
angry after six weeks of hospitalization and new
health threats. Then I was told I was too demanding. Serious errors were made in my timed medication; diuretics were dispensed along with sleep-
ing medication. Because of a stupid computer
error, I was told the cyst on the brain was malignant. I became hysterical and thought, My God!
Everyone had betrayed me—my husband, my doctors—and I've probably got only two or three
weeks left to live. I'll never be released.

My hysteria was so bad, I was sedated, but only
after I was admonished for overreacting after the
error had been corrected. But the sedation caused
me to hallucinate and I know I was wild with rage
. . . and then a psychiatrist was called in to see why
I was upset. I won't tell you what his label for me
was, but boy! I wanted to throw him out of my
room.

How could they be so insensitive and not understand my situation? I mean these were professional caregivers, not unskilled day laborers. Anyway, I apologized again, calmed down, accepted the blame for overreacting, got "whipped into place," and went home to recuperate. My private room cost us $230 a day for forty-one days. The total of all the bills during that illness reached $40,000.

Despite enormous amounts of money that we don't have and all my bad experiences, I'm alive, very happy, and well . . . and that makes it okay that some doctors call me demanding, pushy, intrusive, and aggressive. But I wonder if they realize that as patients, we must muster all our inner resources to put up the fight for life?

I save my questions for each specialist. Then when I get there, they misjudge my concern as being a preoccupation with cancer and an inability to cope.

My case may be unique, but since I'm regarded as a patient advocate who gently informs, not alarms people, I'd like it very much if I was treated accordingly.

Today the technological advancements are phenomenal, but unfortunately our human skills and compassion have not kept pace with them. Nathan Hale may have felt he had but "one life to give," but I don't. I've fought too many bloody battles to quit fighting until there is no spirit left in my cancer-scarred body.

I felt better when I finished writing it. Then I filed the letter in my "sad and mad" file, until now.

Of course, writing isn't the only way to work through anger. Telling a trusted friend or counselor can help. Some people go to a private place to yell, swear, cry, or stamp their feet. Know you're angry, know why, and decide on a method of expression that will work best for you.

One woman told me that her friends had told her to "get angry and fight back" after she was diagnosed with breast cancer. This confused her because she was cheerful, easygoing, and soft-spoken. Although she had faith in her oncologists and had a good prognosis, she began to worry that if she didn't fight back she wouldn't survive.

Becoming mean and hostile is not what is meant by fighting back. Fighting back means rolling with the punches, the ups and down—relishing the good days, doing whatever is necessary to get through the rough days, even if it's crying or watching TV all day. It means a new awareness of life, asking questions when you have doubts, and taking care of your body by doing everything within your power to stay alive.

Often anger can work for you. Constructive anger can be an ally, motivating you and pushing you toward recovery. Many prosthetic devices in use today, I was surprised to learn, were conceived, developed, or improved upon by patients who were angry with products they found inadequate.

Constructive anger pushed me into creating Cancer Call-PAC and developing a better way to prevent my wig from slipping. So don't just complain about something you're dissatisfied with; instead, devote your thoughts and energy to changes that could be made. You never know when that opportunity might arise.

ILLNESS AND GRIEF

This is not a book on death and dying, but grief has a role in any illness, and we find it impossible not to consider the issue. In fact, there are many losses that require a period of mourning.

Any major change, no matter how welcome, involves some kind of loss. People who move, for example, are separated from their neighborhood, friends, and familiar life patterns. A high school graduation, a wedding, a new job—all are accompanied by a slight melancholy, a saying good-bye. Will not illness, then, an unwelcome change, bring with it a sense of grief?

Consider the losses. You lose your well self. You lose much of your lifestyle through adaptations to a new regimen of medical care. Sometimes you lose a part of your body through surgery. Sometimes you lose normal body function that must be recaptured or compensated for in another way.

The impact of each loss is a very individual matter. Some women, for example, seem barely affected by the removal of a breast; they are much more worried about the malignancy. Others report that coping with the loss of a body part gives them their greatest difficulty. Some felt depressed for a few weeks; others say that, months after their surgery, they suddenly weep for no apparent reason. "The world," one patient said, "looks gray; there's no color at all."

However powerful its impact, grief commonly involves sadness (weeping), depression (difficulty making decisions and reengaging in activity), and anxiety (feeling a heightened sense of worry but being unable to grasp about what). Often people cannot cope with the most ordinary tasks. This paralysis does not last—you will feel better eventually—but it does have a purpose: to focus on the work of grief.

After a death, society provides activities to help mourners deal with their loss. Family and friends visit to express their sympathy and to share memories. Funeral and burial arrangements must be made. You don't *feel* like doing anything, but social pressure dictates certain actions. Completing them begins the process that will enable you to continue on your own afterward.

After a major change or loss or illness, however, society is not always so adept. Quite often the opposite happens. Visitors to a hospital bedside may say, "Why are you crying? You're going to be fine." If you remain listless for a period of time, they may start looking for ways to cheer you up—whether you want it or not! And if enough people tell you that you should not feel bad, you may begin to feel worse, wondering, What's wrong with me? If you are not sure of the source of your feelings, ask a wise friend or trusted counselor to help. Think about what losses you have suffered and make a list. Let yourself grieve. Know that your tears are neither unexplained nor unjustified. Struggling to hold them back will only exhaust you. A good cry helps the process, will probably help you rest, and will certainly release energy for other things.

Talk about it. Again, close friends, trusted counselors, patient/family support groups, telephone listening services all are good resources.

Review previous losses in your life. How did you grieve? Can you apply some of the same methods now? Some patients have found physical exercise a help. Others, after the first, most severe period of mourning is over, seek out new, positive activities. One woman, recovering from surgery for a recurrent cancer, decided with her friends that she had had enough bad news for the year and organized a party for the family dog! Sound silly? Maybe, but it helped.

Remember that grief is a process. The periods of sadness will gradually become shorter and further apart. Oddly enough, fighting the process only makes it take longer. Working through your grief will help your recovery.

Is there such a thing as too much grief, mourning that goes on too long? This is a very difficult question to answer, because individual reactions to loss vary so dramatically. Ask yourself if the process "feels" right to you. Or do you sense that the same intensity of sadness, or of dysfunction, has gone on longer than you think it should? If so, talk with a counselor or join a patient/family group; its members can help by affirming a wide range of responses to loss and by sharing their coping strategies.

After a move, you miss your old home, but soon you make new friends, learn a new neighborhood, find new shops. When your hair grows back, it's not exactly like the hair you had, but slowly it becomes more and more a part of what you experience as you. If you wear a breast form, it gradually becomes second nature to insert the form in your bra. And, as you gradually recover from the effects of treatment, you think of yourself less and less as a sick person who has lost a normal life and more and more as a person for whom illness is one experience—but not the only one.

Because we are capable of treasuring life, we are vulnerable to the pain of separation and loss. Grieving is tough, but we do survive. Our reward for seeing the process through is a renewed ability to embrace the treasures of a world that, once again, looks beautiful.

BE KIND TO YOURSELF

The two questions I most frequently am asked are:

"What do you find to smile about when you've been sick so much?"

"Since your life has been threatened, why do you continue to be so involved in helping sick people? Why don't you just go out and have fun?"

My response to both questions is that I've always been optimistic and productive. Finding a fulfilling purpose in life has enabled me to draw on personal talents, and when I'm busy and creative, I'm happy. I'm fortunate that I'm able to do all the things I enjoy doing, so that I'm not bored and dwelling constantly on dying. I don't feel that I'm just living. I feel that I'm very much alive.

Patients preoccupied with illness and treatment often wonder how they could possibly consider participating in enjoyable activities, but engaging in things that brought pleasure before is an adaptive measure and a necessary means of maintaining self-esteem.

Don't give up on life; do things that please you. Activity, whether it's knitting, golfing, playing cards, or singing in a choir, can be a buffer against life's frustrations.

I love writing and reading, and I spend almost every minute I wait in doctors' offices and examination rooms doing what brings me the most fulfillment. Since frequent appointments are a way of life for me, I don't resent the waiting so much because I'm using the time in a creative way.

Some people criticize a patient's attempt to have fun in the midst of serious illness, but caregivers understand that maintaining enjoyable pursuits can alleviate emotional stress. Family members must also be encouraged to resume their pleasurable activities.

At a recent lecture, a young woman in the audience said she was terribly distraught because her mother had lung cancer and she didn't know what to do to help.

She was married and had small children. Her husband had bought tickets to a play she was eager to see, but now that the event was only a week away she felt she should not go.

She cried: "How can I even consider going out for a good time when my mom is so ill with cancer? It's my duty to be with her day and night."

I replied, "Why should you not try to enjoy yourself? Your mother will probably be relieved to see that her illness has not caused you to forgo your own family life. And you will be refreshed, ready to give her the support she does need when she needs it."

GETTING HELP

A safe, comfortable place to turn to for guidance and direction is a hospital's Family Services Department. The staff is equipped to deal with medically related crises, and certainly problems that arise within a family as they struggle through cancer fall into that category. Another source is the hospital's Department of Pastoral Care.

I advocate guidance centers and hospital chaplains because psychiatric therapy usually extends over a long period of time, time the patient may not have. A family waiting in the surgical lounge usually is filled with fear and needs immediate short-term intervention. Many people expect the worst, and too often they get it. When the doctor says, "It's cancer," their world is shattered, and some never move beyond that moment in time.

Hospital Chaplains

Hospital chaplains are pastoral counselors trained in theology and psychology; they are skilled both in crisis intervention and in providing long-term care. Most are religiously affiliated but are not assigned to a parish.

What I particularly appreciate about those I know is that they don't threaten or admonish you for what you are and for what you are feeling. Since we all deal with grief in our own way, chaplains respect such differences by trying to listen to each person carefully. They can't change what already has happened but try to walk with the person or family through their difficulty.

Some people rely on their faith in God to cope with their grief, but others question their faith in times of crisis. Listening is crucial to these chaplains so that their words are appropriate to the situation and not an additional anguish.

The chaplain is available to everyone in the hospital. Patients terrified of impending surgery can talk with the chaplain to identify and work through their fears. And the chaplain will almost never respond with, "Come on, you're a big boy. Stop being so frightened," or "It's God's will."

Later, when the patient is in surgery, the chaplain will comfort the waiting family for which every minute is an eternity. While chaplains aren't perfect, they are best known for the empathy they provide. They don't pass judgment, lecture, scold, or say "I told you so."

When a team of neurologists came to say they were scheduling brain surgery for me, I was astonished and terrified. I also was furious at the casual way they told me.

I was alone, with only a group of doctors and residents staring at me. I was too embarrassed to cry and didn't know how I was expected to respond. So when I caught my breath, I meekly asked, "When?"

"Thursday. Have your husband call me."

When they left the room, I screamed. I didn't know that my daughter had come right from school and had heard every word outside my room. Luckily, a chaplain came on the scene. He understood that I was angry, afraid of surgery, and afraid of dying. He listened and empathized. We cried together, and this helped us so much. Then I prepared to tell my husband the frightening news.

Too often people are unaware of the role of chaplains, and if they've been a bit lax in practicing their religion or attending services, they fear they'll be reprimanded, so they usually say no when asked if they would like to see a chaplain.

But chaplains do not promote membership in any particular faith community. They strive to provide support according to the special needs of each patient they meet.

8
Patient and Family Together

FAMILY LIFESTYLE: NORMALCY OR LUNACY?

Bud: Patients want nothing more after their treatment is completed than a return to normalcy—going back to work, playing golf, rejoining the bridge club—restoring themselves and their families to their previous routine. It gives them confidence that all is right with their world, no matter how chaotic it might be.

What passed for normalcy at our house might be considered lunacy at someone else's. Working in network news means almost never being able to say, "I'll be home for dinner."

The hours are long, but the real problem is that they're unpredictable. A breaking news story could send me from one end of the country to the other without notice and keep me there indefinitely. Middle-of-the-night phone calls ordering me to hop on the first plane out were commonplace. The news does not wait, and those of us in the business become captives of the stories we cover.

Who knows how many dinner dates have been canceled, how many birthday parties have been missed, how many tickets to the theater or opera have gone unused? My friend Ike Pappas who was with CBS, missed the christening of one of his children because he was called in to cover a major story on that day. I was one of his guests at the reception and felt guilty because I hadn't been called in.

I had almost missed our daughter's christening several years earlier because the civil rights riots in Chicago and the Richard Speck murders happened one after the other. We had been working around the clock on those stories, and it was not until literally the last hour that I knew I would be able to take off for the ceremony and reception.

It's something we live with and try to make the most of. Often I would take Geo and the kids with me on an assignment if I knew I was going to be gone for a while and if it was one in which they would not be in the way. That kept our periods of separation down and created a sense of sharing in each other's life that we still have.

My unconventional schedule (by most people's standards) was not too difficult to contend with before Geo became ill. In fact, it was rather exciting. Once, when I had to cover a flood in North Dakota, I called Geo and asked if she wanted to come along. An hour later she had the kids bundled up, and off we went. How many wives can say their husbands took them to see a flood?

When cancer entered our lives, it brought with it a sense of fear and delivered a powerful blow to Geo and to all of us as well. The diagnosis of the disease, along with the medical procedures, surgical scars, and therapy side effects, disrupted our lifestyle, created uncertainty about the future, and caused financial upheaval.

I'll never forget the day Geo came home from the hospital. It should have been a happy day . . . at least happier than those we'd had since Geo underwent surgery. But on that day we'd had to call a repairman to fix the stove, which, displaying a sense of perversity, chose that particular time to break down.

As I helped Geo into the house, we both sensed a state of confusion. The repairman was there. Jimmy, elated that his mother was coming home, was in a state of high excitement but had been admonished to "behave." He darted from the house, fell down, and gashed his knee so badly I had to rush him to the emergency room for stitches.

Meanwhile, friends and neighbors were coming by to say hello. The house was like the Hilton Hotel, doors opening and closing, people coming and going, coffee-pots brewing, the phone constantly ringing, the repair-man crawling around the kitchen, asking us to pass him his tools. That day, I suppose, filled with confusion and conflicting priorities, was good training for the ones that followed.

I don't think there is any prescribed way to deal with a crisis. Even those who are not encumbered by crip-pling or energy-sapping illness find it hard to think their way through crises such as a job loss or problems with their children. For those in physical pain or whose schedules are centered around doctors' visits or medi-cal treatment, problems, the everyday variety and the exceptional, are much more difficult to deal with.

Advice, of course, is plentiful, not only from profes-sional advice givers but from friends, relatives, and strangers as well. But advice, even from qualified and trustworthy professionals, often is contradictory and, more often than not, difficult or impossible to follow. In a flood, does one try to plug the hole in the dike or rush to save his belongings and find a place safe from the water?

Geo's illness had to be dealt with. I was not going to risk her chances of survival by following a pattern of benign neglect—either mine or her doctor's. She was fighting cancer with an uncommon courage. She was bearing her pain with too much cheerfulness to be done in by inattentiveness or out-of-place priorities. It was not hard to make the decision that my first priority was to do everything possible to give her a fighting chance.

But that was not the only matter I had to deal with. A multitude of others had to be addressed, all of them important enough to require a full measure of attention, each of them becoming more complex and sensitive as a result of Geo's illness: the children, my job, finances, our mothers, both of them widowed and needing help. Not uncommon problems by any means, but each, in its way, required more time and energy than I or we had left to give. I felt as though I were watching a motion picture of my life, sitting in front of a movie screen, watching it go by, wanting to change the action but not being able to stop the projector.

Some things sound so simple. You have a problem, you go to the doctor. But going to the doctor is debilitating in itself. Many times I had to take the day off or go to work late so that I could drive Geo to the hospital or to her doctor's office. And many times we would wait for hours because the doctor had been called away to surgery or otherwise delayed. Many times we were shuttled around from office to office until someone decided that his specialty was the one that fit the problem. This process is so draining on both the patient and the person with the patient that it's no wonder many people decide to forgo it, preferring the risk of serious harm to the hassle and discomfort of seeking medical care. What was expected to be a two- or three-hour procedure, including the time it took to go back and forth, often stretched into five or six hours or more, requiring adjustments everywhere down the line.

Would the person watching the children be able to stay a few hours longer than planned? Would the children sense something was wrong? Would they think that their mother wasn't going to be back at all? Would your employer be patient? Would the project you're working on get along without you? When might your employer decide he can get along without you? These are questions you cannot escape when you have an illness that will not go away. They complicate your life and cloud your mind and distract you from the full-time job of trying to stay alive.

The situation is even worse when patients are their families' breadwinners. If their physical condition restricts their ability to perform their jobs, they may find themselves out of work or working at something else for less money. Unless the family has unlimited financial resources (and the majority of families do not), it can result in serious trouble. Homes may have to be sold or will be lost when mortgage payments cannot be met; families are forced to move in with relatives, uprooting everyone; college plans must be scrapped; bills remain unpaid, and credit ratings are affected. Financial disaster is frequently the result.

STAYING IN TOUCH: HUSBAND AND WIFE

Geo: What changed at home following my initial diagnosis primarily was the atmosphere: less laughter, less time for fun, no money for extras or eating out, no more vacations, less time to pursue hobbies. You no longer do things that cost money with friends, such as going to plays or away for a weekend. Their life is moving on while yours seems to be going in reverse because of the medically related expenses. Eventually, they don't extend invitations anymore, so you feel left out. Cutbacks were made across the board, and that included a bag lunch for Bud rather than eating out with friends.

Bud's job changed only by demanding more of his time and attention as major stories broke as never before.

Bud and I agreed that we would not undermine each other and I would handle the day-to-day decisions. Even though I was frequently hospitalized, I was still more accessible to the children than Bud was. I, at least, was only a phone call away.

Easy to do? Absolutely not! It meant that no matter

how sick I was, I couldn't back away from whatever decisions had to be made, and I constantly had to arrange and rearrange plans.

This worked out fine, but over the years a pattern seemed to develop. Bud felt left out of things when he was around. I guess it's like reading a comic strip only on Sunday while others read it every day. You basically have an idea of what is happening but not as detailed an account as if you read it daily.

Bud felt that the children were ignoring him.

I suppose traveling salesmen experience this when they come home and their wives try to update them on what has happened. It's not the same as being there for the daily discussions and decisions. I think I can understand why they feel left out.

One crucial factor that did *not* change for us is our love, trust, and respect for one another. No matter how bad things were, no matter how much stress there was between us, we never contemplated a separation or a divorce. Our marriage was for keeps, and we were determined to see that it lasted forever.

There's not one thing I wouldn't do for Bud, and I know that he feels the same way about me. We are very supportive of each other. I'd push to get well fast so that he wouldn't worry, and he'd hang in there because he knew I needed him.

Bud and I prized the time we had together, and we were determined not to go our separate ways because of his unusual hours. We followed his schedule, and we included the children. We lived a block away from their elementary school, and since their classes began at nine they didn't have to get up until eight. Even if they got to bed at eleven the night before, they were able to get their proper rest.

I always wait up for Bud and always get up with him, whatever the hour. He needs to unwind before he goes to bed, so we usually have a snack, sometimes at one or two in the morning, read awhile, or watch television until he can fall asleep. We average only four or five hours of sleep a night, a pattern that began when we were first married. On his days off, though, we take the phone off the hook, sleep late, and have breakfast in bed.

This is a somewhat goofy schedule, and we've been unable to break it even on vacations. We've been known to drive until eleven at night before pulling into a motel, and while other travelers would be on the road early, we wouldn't hit it until noon or even later.

We've made breakfast our special time together because Bud works through the late news and doesn't get home for supper. And this routine has continued even though the children are grown.

We use the time to talk over *everything*—children, friends, problems, joys. We know that, no matter what the crisis, couples must face it together or, sadly, suffer separately.

One of my hospital roommates was a young woman, very ill with breast cancer. Her husband arrived early every day and stayed late, just sitting quietly beside her. Hospital staff streamed in and out, exchanging pleasantries. He was very talkative with them—but not with his wife. Whenever she dozed off, he told me how badly he wanted to speak with her about her impending death. And after he left at night, she would share her anger and disappointment with him for wasting precious time. I frequently left the room to go to the chapel, hoping the couple would use the opportunity to talk with each other. But they didn't, and she passed away without a word being exchanged between them.

Another young patient I know sought pastoral assistance to cope with her disease. She had recently lost a sister and mother to breast cancer and felt overwhelmed by her diagnosis. Her husband, having been the most important person in her life up to that point, deeply resented his wife's need for emotional support from some other source. Unable to sort through his feelings of hopelessness, despair, and anger, he let her know how rejected he felt, then withdrew completely.

Why do these couples—and others like them—let cancer drive such a wedge in their relationship? What is so fearful about the crisis that they dare not name it? In every case, there is probably a different answer. But whatever the particular worry, Bud and I know that the only way to ease fears is to face them together.

Patients should not be harsh with their loved ones if they temporarily pull away. If they were loving and attentive before diagnosis and treatment, they probably won't change, but they may need time to deal with their own fears and anxieties before they can be supportive.

Expect that the patient and spouse/lover will not have identical feelings; every person reacts differently under stress. But it is important that you share how the experience affects each of you.

Many male patients fear that they'll lose their masculinity and that their mate will no longer care for them. But that's not true in most instances. If you're under treatment and are experiencing a lot of weakness and other side effects, consider how you looked and felt when you had a severe case of the flu and had similar symptoms. Did your mate leave you then because you were wiped out? Or did he or she help nurse you back to better health?

Women shouldn't withdraw from their partners either. Far too many assume their mates will leave them if they lose a breast, so they pull away to spare themselves anticipated emotional hurt.

Patients should remember that their spouse hurts too. Spouses and lovers should remember that patients still need to be needed and don't want the illness to prevent them from playing a supporting role.

To the degree that it's possible, maintain your normal level of intimacy. If you're worried that your partner is too weak or too ill, *ask*; otherwise your loved one may misinterpret your actions, believing they signal withdrawal rather than concern.

Think about how you faced other crises together. How did you respond? Is cancer any different?

If both parties understand what is happening to their lives, they may become even closer.

Schedule private time and don't let anything interfere—not the phone, not the kids, not unexpected company.

And last, remember that it takes time for both parties to get used to the reality that one of them now has a life-threatening illness.

STAYING IN TOUCH: THE CHILDREN

Whether you're the patient or a family member, set ground rules, then make sure they're adhered to. Don't let others make crucial decisions for you. No matter how difficult it might be, it's your life that's at stake, so you'd better be in charge. What might work for others could be totally inappropriate for you. And this applies especially to your relationship with your children.

Don't let reversals interfere with what has to be done. Define your priorities and then hang on to them. No matter what popped up, I'd try as hard as possible not to let anything change what I had decided to do, particularly where Jim and Kerry were concerned. Often I had to postpone plans for a period of time, but I never canceled anything. Birthdays were sometimes celebrated several weeks late, but at least they were celebrated.

If kids are expected to help out more at home, if money for extras isn't going to be available, if it's going to be difficult to allow your children to have their friends play at your home, let them know that there are new rules for now. You can discuss them more or relax them later.

Expect that kids will try to stretch the limits on all the rules you set down. Expect them to tell you their friends can do or go wherever they want.

Expect that the kids will go off by themselves because they need space. Expect that children will resent being "different" and having to do without. Expect that they'll complain about not having designer clothes, trips, etc. But don't get pulled in by these ploys. All parents experience this. All parents feel guilty that they can't give their kids more. Keep remembering it's not just sick parents who are barraged with requests from unhappy teenagers.

Our son, Jim offers the following advice to parents:

- If you can't pinpoint what's causing troublesome behavior, set limits, then deal with each issue as it arises.
- Don't allow one child's problems to overshadow everyone else's needs within the family.
- Get on with the business of living.
- If kids are going to rebel, it's better for it to happen while they are living at home so that parents are able to set limits.
- *Be consistent.*

If you have small children, decide early on if you want to tell them about an illness and be constant about your decision once it's made. Don't be swayed because friends or outsiders tell you to do it differently.

I had tried my best to prepare the children for my absences from home. Things were happening so fast, however, that each homecoming was met with mixed emotions. Our joy and relief were overshadowed by the prospect of repeated separations as I returned to the hospital for more cancer surgery and more treatments.

Since I had made my decision to fight the disease, I had no choice but to go on the roller coaster ride, dragging my husband and small children along.

In an effort to survive, we clung to each other. But every little setback, like a row of dominoes, toppled us all. If I didn't feel well, the children turned to Bud for attention. If Bud was called in to work, their attention reverted to me. Sick or not, I had to take up the slack.

The circumstances drained us emotionally because we drew our strength from each other. But we agreed that since Bud had no control over his work hours, we'd cherish the time we had together. Similarly, though, I had no control over my hospitalization. I'd make sure that the children had as much continued contact with me as possible.

Because Bud's work kept him very busy, I was the constant in Jim's life, and I had a lot of free time to be with him and later with Kerry also. We had been married for four years before we adopted Jim, and we were ready and eager to be parents.

When I became ill, everything in our house changed radically, and it affected Jim even more than I realized at the time, much more so than Kerry, who was only two years old. He became cranky and uncooperative with others and responded only to me.

One of my harshest memories of that early time was when Jimmy entered the Cub Scouts. His den had a rule that one of the parents had to accompany their son to meetings, and the people in charge enforced it with the full authority of Moses handing down the Ten Commandments. Jim had a rough time in scouting because he was always being reminded that his mother was not putting in as much time as other mothers were and that he could not be given special treatment just because his mother was sick. If Bud was working and I couldn't go, he missed out. He did not enjoy Cub Scouts and eventually dropped out, making a number of mothers and scout masters very happy.

A parent's illness affects children in many ways.

Jim was more attached to me than anyone realized and couldn't stand the thought of losing me. He was experiencing terrible anxiety. No matter how articulate children and adults are, they often cannot verbalize anxiety. They just suffer from it.

Kerry already was toilet-trained, but when I was hospitalized she went back to wearing diapers, allowing only Bud or me to change them. She'd go all day

long with a wet diaper, if someone else was watching
her, until one of us was around to change her. Since Bud
went from work directly to the hospital, he'd get home
quite late, but Kerry still would be awake waiting for
him to change her and tuck her into bed.

After my surgery, when I was unable to lift her, she'd
climb onto her dressing table holding a clean diaper, lie
down and wait for me with a big smile on her face. That
became a special time for us.

When I went for radiation every day, Kerry wanted
to come with me and sit quietly for an hour. She didn't
want to stay with her grandmothers or play with
friends. She'd get ready when I did, take her little
purse and dolls, and wait at the door until we left.

She sat outside the isolation room, occupying herself
while she waited for me. Knowing she was there waiting perked me up. In fact, she was usually the only sign
of life in the depressing therapy lounge, since the patients and their families were so despondent.

If I was in the hospital, the children talked with me
daily, and that meant our friends with whom they
stayed also became involved in my physical well-being—cheering up the kids when they were blue, receiving updates on my condition, and finding out when my
test results weren't good. It wasn't easy for many of
them. They were very sincere about helping, but they
couldn't necessarily handle it.

Not everyone can deal with blood and guts or keep
calm in a crisis, so Bud and I began to sort out who
could help us. Some were great about providing rides,
others with shopping and cooking, and still others with
caring for the children.

When I went to Mayo, we had no idea how long we'd
be there, but we knew we had to make the best possible
arrangements for Jim and Kerry at a home where
routine existed with two parents and children.

Chuck and Pat Coughlin, friends with whom I had
worked at the FBI, took the children the first week we

were at the clinic, and Jim and Kerry did everything they did, even going to church with their three children. Pat told me that the first night she put the children to bed, Kerry (then three) asked if the father of the family would tuck her into bed as her daddy did at night. They spent the second week with other FBI friends, Bob and Mary Senne, again a closely knit family with three children. Luckily for us, we've been blessed with many friends who are concerned, understanding, and sympathetic. This ensured that even when we were separated, our children retained a sense of family routine.

And since we kept in touch by phone and were always honest about what was happening, the children never had to wonder where their mother was or how she was. Imagination can cause much greater anxiety than reality, no matter how painful that reality might seem.

FAMILY STRESS

It is a truism, not yet universally understood, that when illness strikes one member of the family, it strikes them all. Most people recognize the pain suffered by the patient, but they rarely see the emotional strain inflicted on his family unless they've been through it themselves.

While the patient's suffering is easily recognizable, that of the family is not. But everyone is hurting—patient, spouse, children, parents—and they can't always see each other's pain. The family suffers right along with the patient but doesn't get the same kind of support.

In many years of working with Call-PAC, through my lectures and letters to the columns I write, 65 percent of the people I've dealt with have been family members and close friends. This surprised me because I thought patients needed more help. I expected that patients needed more understanding and would want to air their fears with someone they knew had made it. Instead, I heard from their families.

I heard, for example, from a young man who could no longer cope with his wife's illness . . . and from a suburban woman who was bewildered by the sudden withdrawal of her husband, a Hodgkin's disease patient, who refused to talk with family members and friends, preferring to stay alone in his room . . . and from a sixteen-year-old cheerleader who questioned why her mother had stopped hugging her and being her pal. She was sure her mother had had a mastectomy and was trying to hide it from her.

My experience with these callers is not unique. An American Cancer Society staff member I've worked with closely for the past sixteen years reports a similar finding:

> During fifteen years in the Service/Rehabilitation program of the American Cancer Society, I became more of an "expert" on relatives than on patients.
>
> While medical/psychosocial resources focus, appropriately enough, on the person who has developed a malignancy, most of the calls to our agency came from family members.
>
> These relatives were confused, upset, and anxious to do the right thing, often unsure of their role. Yet they almost always framed their questions in terms of patient issues. If I tried to shift the discussion to the caller's needs, I met with great resistance.
>
> However much they experienced spiritual and emotional crises, families usually rejected my suggestion that they seek support. Did they think that only the "sick" person deserved assistance? Were they being offered help of which I was unaware? Did they refuse it? Or did others not perceive their needs?

Haven't we been overlooking something important here? Approximately one million Americans are diagnosed annually as having cancer. And, for almost every new case, there is a spouse or child on whom the disruption, uncertainty, and anxiety has a powerful, potentially destructive impact. For all the psychosocial studies of persons with cancer, relatively little has been published about or for those whose lives are affected directly by the patient's illness. Their problems include:

- Being too deeply involved as caregiver to the patient and unable to set realistic limits on their expectations of themselves.
- Suffering from physical exhaustion if there are only one or two people who can help the patient. They feel guilty and frustrated when they want to do something for themselves or go somewhere besides the hospital.
- Doing too much, unwittingly turning the patient into a semi-invalid even when he or she is ambulatory. Then, if the patient improves, the loved one experiences difficulty in "letting go" and trying to resume his own lifestyle.
- Experiencing continual anxiety when cancer becomes an ongoing illness with no end in sight.
- Feeling totally helpless when they realize how much pain the patient has to endure and that they can't wipe it away. In fact, there isn't much they can do except reassure the patient how much they care.
- Fearing for their jobs. Very few people can rely on the goodwill of their employer to allow unlimited time off for personal business.
- Having extreme difficulty in making decisions. It is a powerful responsibility to assume control on behalf of an unconscious or incompetent loved one.
- Harboring guilt: for being well, for being angry with the one who is ill, for seeking relief.

Some people experience *all* of these problems. They try to maintain their daily routine—going to work or school, doing the laundry, the shopping, the cooking. They visit the patient in the hospital and keep friends and relatives updated. It's a hassle just for a week, and if the patient is hospitalized for five or six, the family can easily fall into a state of exhaustion trying to keep a frantic pace.

They need a break. They need time to rest and replenish their emotional reserves, but they don't get it. And chances are, when the patient leaves the hospital, his or her homecoming is not necessarily met with overwhelming enthusiasm, particularly if the patient needs continuing care at home.

The kind of care provided routinely in the hospital—managing pain and distress, providing meals and medication, changing beds and bandages—cannot be duplicated at home, and the patient may feel that the family is just not trying hard enough. The family, now the primary or only caregivers, may not be making those daily trips to the hospital, but the demands on their time and energy become even greater.

Sometimes caregivers, in a desire to be helpful and accommodating, unwittingly create or perpetuate a situation that is debilitating and unworkable. They have so much to do, both in terms of physical care and in terms of the household tasks once performed by the patient. Juggling their own commitments and the new demands on their time, they can quickly approach burnout. They need permission—even encouragement—to explore alternatives, as long as those alternatives do not lessen the quality of care the patient is receiving. No one person can meet all the physical and emotional needs of another. But when a loved one is ill, the temptation to try can become overwhelming!

Julie (not her real name), a twenty-four-year-old single parent, cried as she told me about her widowed mother, who had had a breast removed.

"I feel so trapped, I don't know how I can ever find a way out." Julie was separated from her husband but continued to live in a far south suburb. When her mother learned she had cancer, she moved in with Julie and her four-year-old son. Julie's mother was receiving daily radiation treatments and insisted on continuing her care at a hospital on the far north side where she had had her surgery.

Julie drove her back and forth, a round-trip of 115 miles that took about five hours every day in an old car that got terrible gas mileage. She quit her daytime job to be available to help her mother and began waitressing at night. Her four-year-old was cranky from the long car ride and the equally long wait at the hospital. When she got home each day at three, Julie had to shop, clean house, and do laundry before she started work at eight. Then she stood at work for eight hours and returned home at 4:00 A.M. She averaged about four hours of sleep a night.

She was exhausted to the point of collapse and felt angry and guilty. She told me she was ashamed to have these feelings since her mother was so ill, but she couldn't imagine continuing such a routine for three more months, and she couldn't bring herself to discuss these issues with her mother.

Before her mother's treatments were completed, she was hospitalized again. This added another burden because Julie now needed a sitter for her son. The expenses for gas, parking, and a sitter almost equaled the salary and tips she got.

"I can't be responsible for everyone. I can't afford it, and I'm worn out," she said, adding that she was angry at herself for being annoyed with her mother at a time when she needed help.

I asked if she could skip visiting her mother for a day or two and spend that time doing something special for herself and Mark. "I'd love to do that," she said, "but do you think I could?" Julie badly wanted to stay home but didn't allow herself to. My mentioning it made it acceptable.

Like many family members, Julie needed to learn how to set limits. Her commitment had become a burden so overwhelming she could no longer cope, yet she could not limit the time and energy given to her mother without experiencing tremendous guilt.

She finally spoke with a chaplain (at my insistence) and called me one week later, elated. After her visit with the chaplain, she had skipped three days of hospital trips, taken her son to the zoo, and gone shopping with a friend. Julie needed "permission" to give herself some time—to recognize and accept her limits and to realize that, in the long run, time out meant more time to give.

When I was diagnosed, my mother, a recent widow, felt guilty, as though it was her fault I had cancer because it is prevalent on her side of the family. Both her husband and mother had died within a week of each other; she was grief-stricken, depressed—not a good candidate to live with us and help me cope with my first round of radiation therapy.

We discussed the options and agreed it made more sense for her to move in with her brother, Father George Thomas, a Greek Orthodox priest. It has worked beautifully. Keeping house for him and becoming involved in parish activities helped her recover from her overwhelming grief. She visits me when I am not taking treatments or in the hospital, for at those times my illness would be too upsetting for her. Instead, she comes for long visits when I am well and we can enjoy our companionship.

FAMILY STRENGTH

Bud: The previous pages may seem like a litany of problems, but they also contain the solutions. If we learned nothing else over the past twenty years, we learned that the only way to deal effectively with family issues is to face them squarely.

Be Clear and Direct

While serious, chronic illness imposes real stresses on family life, the strains *can* be eased if everyone recognizes them and agrees to deal with them together.

Use the Problem to Determine Its Solution

When Geo's illness and my job threatened our time together, we scheduled family time—at odd hours, perhaps, but still family time. When our son Jimmy acted out his fear and confusion by running away from home, we dealt with it by confronting not his behavior but the feelings behind it. After that, he could tell us when he was upset, rather than acting it out.

Make Sure Everyone Participates

When you identify a problem, schedule a family meeting when everyone can be present. You can only do this, of course, if you have decided from the first to be honest about what is happening. The family benefits, however, because each member becomes part of the solution, and the bonds you forged before remain strong.

Make Sure No One Is Overwhelmed

Even with the best of intentions, a busy, stressed family can fail to notice that one of the members is carrying most of the load. Sometimes it's because the family "worker" volunteers for too much; sometimes the most capable member is assigned too much. Whatever the reason, you can usually spot the problem: one member is always tired and may be irritable or withdrawn. If that happens, tackle the problem together. Find out who is responsible for what and reassign tasks as necessary.

Recognize Every Contribution

Geo: Bud often calls me from work—even if for only a few seconds—providing a caring presence that helps me throughout the day. After my brain surgery, Kerry willingly took charge of the house, drove me wherever I had to go, and without complaint, once again postponed going away to school, continuing instead to take courses at a nearby college. When Bud became ill and was forbidden by his physician to drive, Jim provided his transportation when I couldn't. We gained strength, not from attempting to complete our routine chores alone, but through our support of each other.

Don't Keep the Sick Member Confined to That Role

Whoever the patient is—mother, father, daughter, son—that person cannot be allowed (or forced) to drop the family role for that of sick person. I have been wife and mother and cancer patient, but if I had become a patient only, I would have denied Bud and the children their family relationships with me. This is not easy to do: sometimes, as mother, I must discipline my children; as patient, I need their help, and they need to be of help to me.

Make Sure That Coping Time Is Matched by Fun Time

Families struggling with illness can be tempted to remain serious all the time, and that's a mistake. Whatever was fun before will be fun now—try it! Whether it's sports, picnics, games, movies, dining out, or a trip, your family needs and deserves recreation. You don't hesitate to share your sorrows; share your laughter, too.

Expect that your priorities are going to take a healthy jolt. I soon discovered that the medical demands on my time forced me to cut through a lot of unnecessary clutter.

I realized it wasn't important to have the cleanest windows on the block. If I didn't vacuum often, so what? We delayed major spring cleaning for nearly four years. We always kept the house neat and clean—we just didn't have the time and energy to tear it apart, to wash walls and clean carpets, etc.

We converted our bedroom into an all-purpose room, with a television, desk, phone, the kids' toys—everything we needed accessible to us—so that the kids would be near when I had to rest or Bud had paperwork to do.

One year we didn't take our Christmas tree down until May. The children loved it, and that's what counted.

Not attending PTA meetings or making cupcakes for their bake sales may have made me seem uncooperative, but spending valuable time with my children was far more important.

What sustained me was my family and my faith. No matter how bad I felt, I made daily visits to church. Everything else often got short shrift—and rightly so.

Part Three
WHAT YOU CAN DO

9
For Those Who Live, Love, Work, and Play with Us

Bud: Lost or strained friendships are heartbreaking but potential side effects of a long-term illness.

Some people simply cannot deal with a good friend's pain. Others are unwilling to invest the time and energy in continuing a relationship that may require more than they are prepared to give.

It's easier for a golf foursome to dump a member who's lost a leg than to find something else they can do together. If that's the way it has to be, then that's the way it has to be.

Patients will mourn the loss of your friendship, may even resent it, so don't make it worse by making excuses: "I really like the guy, but he'd only slow us down." It's bad enough your friend has lost a leg; don't blame him for breaking up your foursome.

Nearly everyone rallies for the first crisis. But as time goes by, some weary of the situation and return to their own interests, their own lives; the attention of the

affected family, however, is repeatedly drawn back to
the recurrent demands of chronic disease.

When 1½-year-old Jessica McClure fell into a Texas
well, the nation watched, riveted, as rescue efforts
progressed. The happy ending came within days. But
who supports the athlete paralyzed in an accident? Who
continues to visit, write, call, as the days become weeks,
then months, then years? Only the most stalwart of
friends.

Never think you can "do nothing" for a friend who is
ill. Those who live, love, work and play with us are vital
to our continued ability to cope. We know! Our friends'
support uplifts us still!

Geo: Many people say they don't know how to act
around their friends who have cancer. A certain
amount of awkwardness is to be expected. But you
haven't changed and your friend hasn't either. Not
really. There are no rules on how to act here, so just be
yourself. Let your intuition guide you.

One way to ease communication is to ask not only
"How are you feeling?" but also "What are you feeling?"
Some people are very willing to talk about their illness
and look for signs that friends are willing to listen.
Others may want to talk one day and not the next, and
still others may never be ready.

What they might need most is someone who doesn't
necessarily "do" anything but allows the patients free-
dom to express their feelings. When I was going
through a rough period, the friends who helped most
were those who went to church with me, hugged me, or
held my hand. Actions can be more important than
words at times like this.

Patients sometimes test those closest to them by asking leading questions such as:

"Has my husband [wife] said anything else to you?"

"Do you know what they're planning to do to me?"

"Have you heard when I'll be able to go home?"

They may be trying to find out if their doctor has told
you the same thing he's told them or if you're going to

lie and pretend their condition is less serious than they already know it is. Sometimes, if they haven't seen their doctor, they may be looking for information, as I was after my first mastectomy when I asked Bud if it was malignant.

The way you answer probably will set the tone for your visit. It will tell the patient if he or she can trust you, if you're going to level with him or her, or if you're going to try to bluff your way through. It's the difference between a helpful visit and one that isn't, one that may not be worth the energy the patient has to expend, one that will make the patient feel worse than before you walked in.

What should you do? For starters, be open and honest, but avoid making gaffes such as one attributed to a reporter interviewing an accident victim in the hospital: "Have they told you they cut off your leg?"

If you have information the patient does not, don't blurt it out. That should come from the doctor, spouse, or someone designated by the family.

But if you do make a mistake, don't dwell on it. Most patients appreciate an empathetic friend, who might say the wrong thing, rather than one who ignores their illness.

No set of guidelines for being a good friend can replace your own style. It's *your* friend, and you know best how your relationship works. However, if you'd like a few simple tips, here they are:

1. Don't be afraid to ask me what I have, how I'm doing, what my treatment will be. At worst, I'll say I don't want to discuss it—and is that so bad? At best, I'll welcome the chance to talk about my situation.

2. Worried about what to say? What did we talk about before I became ill—politics, art, religion, the PTA? I'm still interested. If you're my colleague, let's talk about our work. I'd like to keep in touch.

3. Don't try to cheer me up by telling me things could be worse, that I'm lucky my husband hasn't left, or that I could have been hit by a truck. It doesn't help.

4. In fact, don't try to cheer me up at all. What I need most when I'm depressed is a compassionate comforter.

5. Don't assume you know how I feel. If you're prepared to find out, do ask, for I need every sensitive, empathetic listener I can get.

6. If I look terrible, don't tell me I look "great." Your lie will hang between us and undercut anything else you say. You don't have to comment on my looks at all.

7. Remember, I chose my doctor, and unless I say otherwise, I'm probably satisfied with him. Don't bring me articles about other doctors, other hospitals, other treatments, unless I ask you to.

8. Do bring flowers, books, games—whatever you know I like. Most of all, bring yourself. Illness interrupts so much—*don't* let it interrupt our friendship.

9. When visiting at the hospital, try to be sensitive to the situation. Be alert to my need to talk or to rest, to visit with you, or to listen while you visit with others.

10. When I first come home from the hospital (or after radiation or chemotherapy), I may look good, but I'll be exhausted. I won't have the energy for long visits, either on the phone or in person. Also, just because I'm confined to the house doesn't mean I have the strength to baby-sit for you; don't ask me to.

11. Encourage but don't push my steps toward recovery. I tire easily. They may be small steps . . . remember, though, I can still use a large cheering section!

12. If anything about my illness troubles you, if it makes you upset, or sad, or nervous—tell me! Your silence may hurt me, something I know you don't want. We are friends; let's work it out *together*.

The encouragement of friends helps patients realize that they have not changed simply because they have cancer. Your support may give them the courage to resume their former activities and return to as normal a life as their illness permits.

Just before Bud and I left for Mayo in 1969, we received an excited phone call from our dear friends, Andy and Sia Callas, who announced the birth of their son, Chris. We were to be his godparents, and they assured us that they wouldn't schedule his baptism until we could be there.

It gave me a tremendous lift that, in spite of my illness, I would still be included. And when I returned home, even though I was very ill, the christening preparations gave me something to look forward to.

WHATEVER YOU DO, *DON'T* . . .

I've had some wonderful help and support over the years, but I also have been told or have overheard some pretty tasteless, damaging, and inaccurate comments.

Some people do it in ignorance. Others blurt out their own fears, projecting them onto an unsuspecting patient. Whatever the reason, their effect can be devastating. Here are a few terrible, but true, examples:

1. Many women with breast cancer have told me that other women remarked, "How awful—to have cancer and to have to worry about losing your husband, too." Inconsiderate? Of course. It's also wrong. While it's normal to worry about how a loved one will react to a change in your body, the fact is that most men do not respond negatively to the loss of a breast. They are much more concerned with the health of their wives than with a change in their wives' appearance.

2. At a party, a man who had heard Bud's wife had been ill presumed she had died and said to me, "You must be the second Mrs. Photopulos."

3. Another time, at a restaurant with several other couples, we pushed the table closer to the chairs. "Wait a minute," one woman said. "Just because Georgia's had her breasts removed doesn't mean we all have the same problem." I know it was meant as a joke, that she meant nothing cruel, but it didn't come out that way.

Think before you talk!

4. When we were ordering carpeting for our den, the salesman recognized me from a recent television show and called my husband aside to give him some advice.

"Why don't you wait and see if she makes it. You could be wasting your money now. A new wife might not have the same taste, and you'd have to recarpet the room again. Know what I mean?" This man assumed I would die, didn't realize that Bud would be offended by his remarks, and apparently thought that the cost of a carpet was more important than my survival!

5. A number of years ago, when we sold the home we loved and had lived in for seventeen years, we felt its close proximity to schools, churches, and neighborhood shops would be a strong selling point, perfect for a family with young children. Realtors told us, however, that while their clients loved the house, they would not buy a home previously occupied by a cancer patient.

Incidents like these occur more often than you might think. They can be traced to two things: fear of cancer and the mistaken belief that cancer is contagious. Cancer is *not* contagious. Unfortunately, fear and superstition are.

6. When I began my first bout with cancer, and family pressures began to show, one "friend" suggested that we should return our children to the adoption agency since things were so rough. I will never understand what prompted that remark. It made me very angry. Children are not "rented" until things get tough or loved until other issues take their place.

A related and no less upsetting experience is that of recovered patients who are discouraged by friends and agencies from initiating adoption procedures. This happens even when the doctor has written a "clean bill of health" letter. A cancer history should not disqualify someone from adoption—it doesn't disqualify others from having children. Furthermore, the only way to live life to the fullest is to make plans for the future and act on them. Anyone who waits until things are perfect will soon realize there is no perfect time.

7. I've overheard "friends" shut off communication with comments like these:

"Don't tell me you don't feel well; you don't look sick."

"I know just what you mean about medical bills piling up. We haven't finished paying off our vacation to Hawaii yet."

"Don't think about it." That usually means, "I don't want to hear about it."

Some people don't think. Others are misinformed. Still others are so tied up by their own attitudes and fears they assume everyone thinks and feels as they do. After an encounter with one of them, the patient needs extra support from a true friend—like you.

FOR SPOUSES, LOVERS, AND IMPORTANT OTHERS

Bud: Most men I know like to suffer in silence, especially those my age. Okay, maybe they don't like to but they do.

With good reason!

Most of our boyhood heroes—Joe DiMaggio, Joe Louis, Gary Cooper, Charles Lindbergh—were men who said little, rarely let their feelings show, and suffered their pain and sorrow silently, their joys also. Can you imagine DiMaggio throwing a high five after hitting a home run or Louis dancing around the ring after knocking out an opponent? Did either ever say, "I was robbed?"

Movies were filled with what was called the "strong, silent type," men who took the blows without complaint, who won without boasting, who lost without crying. Wars, ballgames, love—it didn't matter. Whatever happened, our hero took it like a man.

The books we read were the same, especially Ernest Hemingway's, his style sparse, efficient, unemotional, underscoring the prevailing view of manhood. Our fathers never let us see them cry, never admitted having pain or sorrow.

Is it any wonder, then, that men of my generation

don't know how to talk about their problems even with their oldest friends? They keep silent, internalizing their feelings until the fear becomes so unbearable they simply cannot suppress it any longer.

Telling men like this that they have to let it out does no good at all. They'll let it out when they're good and ready to let it out, and when they are, their first choice of a shoulder to lean on usually is not one of their old buddies but a woman, maybe a friend's wife, maybe a co-worker, maybe even a stranger. Nothing seductive here, no ulterior motive. Men find it hard to believe that other men will not consider them weak or think of them as wimps. I can't count the number of times a male friend has called me and then said, "Oh, by the way, may I speak to Georgia for a minute?"

It doesn't seem to make a difference whether the male is the patient or whether he's concerned about his loved one. Not long after I wrote this paragraph, an example so typical occurred that I decided to include it:

I received a call from a friend I had not seen or heard from in at least twenty years. My conversation with him lasted less than twenty seconds.

"Bud?"

"Yes."

"This is Fred _____."

"Hi Fred, how're you doing?"

"I've got a tumor."

"Gee. I'm terribly sorry to hear that."

"Can I talk to Georgia?"

Fred cut off the conversation with me immediately.

The same evening we had dinner with another old friend who recently had had cancer surgery. I wanted to ask about it, find out how he was feeling, give him a chance to talk about it, which he had said he wanted. Instead, he started to talk about a basketball game we had played in almost thirty years earlier, one that I could not remember but that was incredibly fresh in his mind. We talked about basketball and baseball games we had played, about politics, about food. Later, he moved over and talked to Georgia about his illness in graphic detail.

It's important to men that they keep up their facade. Letting it fall is a betrayal of all they've been taught. "Don't flinch." "Don't back off the plate." "Keep a stiff upper lip." Still, they know it is simply a facade. They do hurt, they do cry, and there are times when they want to run away. They know it, and they know others know it. But they don't know how to talk about it, and they don't know how to listen to others talk about it. They live by the old army put-down: "Tell it to the chaplain."

Many male friends asked me how I was doing, but few stuck around long enough to hear the full answer because it bothered them. "That's rough," they'd interrupt as they shook their heads sadly, changed the subject, or beat a hasty retreat. Fortunately, a few were brave enough or patient enough not only to ask but to listen.

I remember especially Don and Yanula Stathulis, who would call from Toledo to get an update on Geo's condition. "We want to hear about Georgia," they would say, "but we also are concerned about how you're doing." They gave me a chance to say that I was worried, that I was scared, that I didn't know what I would do if she didn't survive. They didn't say, "I gotta go now," if I got sort of weepy.

Maybe that's the key to the problem. Men don't handle tears well, their own or someone else's, so they walk away before they come.

Women seem to deal with these matters in a much better way. I've heard many say, "I have a good cry then pull myself together and get on with things." Perhaps they've never been told, as men have, that crying is a sign of weakness, or perhaps they understand the therapeutic value of tears. Women tend to deal with personal problems much more directly than men do. They tend to know themselves better—they know their bodies, they know their limits and recognize them sooner—

they are quicker to reach out to friends and talk with them and are quicker to take other action.

These tendencies may be intuitive or they may be the result of the roles women have played—as daughters, wives, mothers, childbearers, comforters. Or maybe, as I suspect, they are not only more sensitive but stronger than men, better able to face calamity and better able to deal with it. But even these qualities do not relieve them of worry, fear, or anxiety—problems we all share.

Let me make some suggestions here. They're written with the generic masculine pronoun but they apply equally to men and women, husbands or wives, sons or daughters, friends of both sexes.

First, if your friend doesn't want to talk about it, don't push him. It won't help. If he does want to talk, don't ask a general question such as "How's it going?" Start by asking how his wife is, what her treatment is, what her prognosis is. *Resist* the temptation to say, "I knew someone who had the same thing." He's not interested, not now anyway.

Ask him if he's getting any sleep, if he's going to work, how much time he's spending at the hospital, if he needs some company, or if you can take him out to eat when he leaves the hospital.

Tell him you care about him and offer to help him, but offer a specific kind of help, like taking the kids to a ballgame with your own.

When our children were small and Geo was so sick, friends took them to pick pumpkins every October, along with their own children. The children loved doing it and looked forward to it every year. I enjoyed the day off, too, because Geo was usually in the hospital during that month.

I remember another time when a colleague, John Oxman, went "above and beyond" by donating blood in my place, not because Geo needed it—she didn't—but because I was too run-down to make my regular donation at the blood bank.

Meet your friend at the hospital for a cup of coffee or

a sandwich. Offer to be there while his wife is in surgery or having an important test when he might be very anxious. But don't make promises you can't keep. And don't immediately offer him money. You may think you're doing him a favor, but you'll only make him feel uncomfortable, perhaps resentful.

Ask instead about his insurance and offer to help him sort his bills and fill out claim forms. If he needs money, you'll find out then, and you can suggest ways to come up with it, including getting loans from friends. And you can always, of course, line up other friends to send cash instead of flowers or candy.

Some of our friends did this when Geo had her brain surgery, and it helped with the bill for her private room that insurance didn't cover completely. We appreciated that act of kindness. *Remember*, this is a very delicate issue. Let the shared experience of your friendship be your guide.

But one more thing: if money is a very serious problem in a long-term illness and you are in a position to help, don't wait until it's too late to do so. Order your friend to put aside his pride and do what is right for his family, just as our friends did with the plane tickets that enabled us to take the children to stay with their aunt and uncle in Florida until Georgia had recuperated. But *please*, don't announce your good deed to the whole world.

Another time Geo received a one-hundred-dollar bill in an unsigned get-well card. That kind act meant a lot to her, and she never forgot it. She analyzed the handwriting on every card she ever received after that, trying to find out who it was. She finally (almost ten years later) discovered the friend who sent it had also had cancer and knew the financial hardships it created.

HELPING THE FAMILY

Geo: When I was given my initial diagnosis on our tenth wedding anniversary, the children were five and two years old. We quickly learned that the pain of a loved one becomes the pain of the family; the hurt of a loved one becomes the family's hurt, too.

Serious illness affects family, friends, and colleagues who, to one degree or another, share its impact. Furthermore, the agendas of other family members are often put aside because all attention is focused on the patient. Family members, though, desperately need their own support base and empathy.

Don't let your natural concern for the patient blind you to the needs of the family. They can use your help, too. Here are some suggestions:

1. Remember that any emotional support you give to a family member is a gift to the patient as well. For example, our dear friends Mary Ann and Bob Barrett allowed us to use their cottage at Lake Geneva because we couldn't afford to go away.

2. Because family members often have a hard time asking for help, don't just say, "Let me know if you want anything." If possible, make a specific offer: "I would like to visit tonight to see how you're doing. Is that a good time?" "I'm going to the grocery store tomorrow; is there anything I can pick up for you?" "We're making soup this week. What would be a good day to bring some over?"

3. Cards, letters, and personal visits keep the patient in touch throughout the illness and let him know he is not forgotten. Cards, letters, and personal visits to the family do the same thing.

4. Transportation can become a major issue, whether it's to take the patient to medical appointments or for household needs. If you can't drive, perhaps you can help organize a transportation pool.

Georgia Booras did just that. She helped in so many ways—and when she couldn't drive me to an appointment, she enlisted one of her friends to take me. An unexpected bonus: I made many new friends this way.

5. Families with small children need lots of trustworthy baby-sitting help. When the patient is in the hospital or away for treatment, children need supervision and a supportive environment. Only good friends or relatives can provide this.

Our neighbor, Laurene Barsi, a teenager, was like a mother's helper to me for quite a few years. The children adored her, and so did we. She was very responsible and reliable. She not only watched the children; she also helped them with schoolwork, took them to the park, and, whenever my appointments ran late, home to dinner with her family.

Sophia Dimoglis, one of my closest friends, was always helpful. Her children went to the same school as ours and were good friends, too. Jim and Kerry often stayed at Sophia's when I was hospitalized. This kept the disruption of the children's schedule to a minimum.

6. Offer to do errands for caregivers or to sit with the patient while the family does them. If the patient is hospitalized, maybe the family needs someone to look after the home, the pets, and mow the lawn, or shovel the snow.

7. Food preparation takes energy, and families in crisis don't have much left. Baked goods, homemade soups, and casseroles are especially helpful. One patient told me that she hadn't cooked for her family in two weeks because caring friends had brought so much.

8. Everyone needs a break. Take a family member to lunch, or the park, or a movie—whatever he or she would like to do.

9. If a family member confides in you, keep it in confidence. If you really think he or she should talk to someone else (the patient, another family member, a counselor?), then say so. Don't talk to a third party without the person's knowledge and consent.

10. If none of these suggestions seems right for the family you know, ask what you can do, and do it.

HOW TO GET THROUGH TO YOUR DOCTOR

Geo: For twenty years we have met, listened to, lectured to, and worked with countless numbers of patients and their families. They've told us things they don't tell their friends, doctors, or counselors.

We've also spoken to hundreds of friends, doctors, and counselors who've told us things they don't tell their patients.

When appropriate, we've tried to facilitate communication between patients and those who care about them. This book provides another opportunity. Let's take the patients first.

Whenever I lecture to medical audiences I am routinely invited to act as a patient advocate. Most professionals genuinely want to know more about their patients' feelings.

Yet, when I speak to the public, there is one question I know I'll be asked: "How can I talk to my doctor?" The corollary is, of course, "How can I get my doctor to listen to me?"

Once I waited five weeks for an appointment with a specialist too busy to answer my questions over the phone. When the big day finally arrived and I had my one-on-one opportunity, he was paged three times during our visit. Then he rushed to an emergency and admonished me for being anxious.

I was hurt and upset. To me, any problems concerning brain abnormalities are terrifying, and I felt I deserved some empathy after the harrowing experience I'd had with the surgery and subsequent meningitis.

Most people don't want to change doctors. But when they do, it's usually because the doctor doesn't listen to them, so they conclude he doesn't care. Brusque and inconsiderate office staff also turn patients away.

There's a big difference between "cancerphobics" or hypochondriacs and thoughtful, concerned patients who plan their appointments carefully, bring written questions, and genuinely wish to be participants in their own care. Doctors can either enroll patients in their mutual effort or, by ignoring them, in effect, send them away.

Many times before beginning a procedure, doctors told me, "This won't hurt." But it did. Sometimes I felt excruciating pain and was angry that I had been misled and hadn't been given the chance to "psych" myself up to tolerate it. On those occasions, the pain was followed by anxiety, and medication didn't do a thing to stop the hurt or to calm me down.

When I was being prepped for radiation, doctors used a gentian violet needle to outline the areas to be treated—my throat, sternum, chest wall, which was still raw and unhealed from surgery and with a lot of scar tissue from previous surgeries for fibrocystic disease. My arms were held up over my head so that my underarms could be marked, and as three technicians hovered over me I was told, "Be still; this won't hurt."

Have you ever had your underarms pierced with a needle? I was afraid, anxious, angry, frustrated, helpless, and terribly intimidated.

I could have accepted the pain more easily if they had said, "This will hurt for a few minutes, but we'll work quickly and try not to hurt you any more than is absolutely necessary."

Another common misunderstanding occurs when doctors downplay surgery or use their own jargon. When a doctor says "open her up," he implies it's as simple a procedure as opening your mouth for the dentist.

Maybe because they do surgery all the time, it's routine for them, but "open 'em up, close 'em up," makes it sound so safe, so simple, so painless, and so risk-free that the bewildered family isn't emotionally prepared when the patient can't go bowling the day after being discharged.

Surgery is a big deal, and so is its follow-up treatment. If the physician soft-pedals the experience too much, a patient may mistakenly think that normal pain or weakness indicates a serious problem.

Some people think cancer diminishes mental ability. It doesn't. Patients hurt when others tell them what to do or treat them as if they were incapable of understanding. They're not—but patients *are* under tremendous stress, which can result in communication problems. These problems can be overcome, however, when the medical staff invests some extra time at the beginning.

One of my readers aptly described it:

> Recently, after four whirlwind days of tests, my father was sent to a neurologist for consultation and possible brain surgery. While a referring physician usually knows the specialist, a patient and family have to take such a referral on faith.
>
> We were anxious about Dad's condition and nervous about delivering him into the hands, however competent, of a stranger.
>
> This particular stranger not only provided competence, but communication.
>
> After Dad's hospital admission, a nurse clinician from the surgeon's practice, who concentrates on patient/family communication, told him that after the team's review was completed, a family-and-friends conference would be scheduled and my father could notify those he wanted to attend.
>
> We were given a complete summary of the tests performed, their results, and shown the film studies. The surgical proposal included the risks and benefits, and everyone had a chance to ask questions.
>
> It might have been "easier" for the surgeon to visit my father alone, declare the necessity for surgery, and depart. Instead, the team did a more difficult thing—spent time and energy with a room full of very distraught people. What a positive difference that made!

1. The conference put the patient in control of the information flow.

2. It allowed my father to enjoy the support of those who love him at the time he needed us most. And we had the energy to give it, because we weren't distracted by trying to find out what was happening.

3. It saved time. The team didn't have to answer the same questions from many different people—and how would the physician have known who had my father's permission to be involved?

4. It made him a better surgical risk. Knowledge reduces anxiety.

5. During the operation, the nurse clinician kept us informed of every step. The presurgical conference helped us understand these reports.

6. Several days were required before all the studies could be completed, but we waited quite easily. We knew when the findings would be given and who would give the report.

I think the information conferences made us all more effective members of the health care team. They allowed the surgeon to concentrate on his skill, the nurse clinician to exert her communication talents effectively, the patient to focus on the challenge he faced, and his family and friends to contribute emotional support.

Of course we had moments of anxiety, of tears, of anger; and we were supported, in turn, by an excellent, caring nursing staff.

Wouldn't it be marvelous if all health professionals conducted their practices in the same manner?

The same woman also told me how the health care team helped the family with a good blend of honesty and hope.

Before the craniotomy we were told the surgery was very serious, but we hoped that he would come through it well and that the tumor would be a lymphoma, which is very responsive to treatment.

He did survive the operation, but they found a
rapidly growing, incurable cancer. We hoped for a
remission with radiation therapy; it did not work.
Then we hoped he would be pain-free—and he
was—and that he would be able to die at home, and
he did. We always knew exactly what was happening, yet we always had *something* to hope for.

PERFECT SUPPORT—IMPERFECT RESULTS

Personal value systems, whether based on religious
conviction, ethnic background, or cultural heritage, are
hard to dislodge, even in times of crisis. In fact, the
patient may rely on them even more.

If advice—no matter how sensible—conflicts with
these values, it will not be taken. When someone you
know refuses treatment and you know this refusal will
cost a life, it's frustrating, but it's *not* your fault, and no
matter how painful it might be for you, you can't do a
thing about it.

I've talked with many patients who failed to pursue a
treatment course. Here's a sampling:

- A twenty-one-year-old exchange student whose
  faith community did not believe in blood transfu-
  sions. A leukemia patient, she was caught between
  her fear of the disease and her fear of rejection by
  her family and similarly convinced friends.
- A forty-two-year-old widow whose husband had
  drowned on a camping trip. She was found to have
  a metastasis several months after his death. Her
  ten-year-old twin sons, who had witnessed their
  father's drowning, were still in shock. She refused
  the recommended adrenalectomy because she felt
  her children could not handle an extended separation from her so soon after the loss of their father.
- A nurse from the Philippines, working in a big city

in the United States, found a large lump in her breast but refused to see a doctor. Her family had pooled its resources to send her to the United States to become a nurse so that she could earn money to eventually bring the rest of her family here. She felt this financial responsibility deeply, and since she wouldn't be paid a full salary on extended sick leave, she elected to forgo treatment and keep working.

- A middle-aged man being treated for an ulcer by a doctor who also was his brother-in-law. While the doctor was on an extended visit to Europe the patient collapsed, was taken to a hospital, and was found to be suffering not from an ulcer but from stomach cancer. Afraid of offending his family, he refused treatment until his brother-in-law returned a few months later, even though he had been warned that delay would be fatal.

All of these patients died without revealing to anyone else *why* they refused treatment. But even if they had shared their reasons, we cannot know whether they could have been persuaded to change their minds.

To many people, some things are more important than life itself. However, they still need you for supportive care. Knowing that you disapprove of their decision, they may be afraid to ask for it.

You may be afraid that your supportive care will imply that you agree with this decision. If you become troubled, talk to a responsible professional, like a hospital chaplain, who can help you sort out the conflicting values involved.

Sometimes patients suffer from much more than the illness, something their friends or doctors do not know and can't be expected to know.

I received a call from an angry forty-seven-year-old woman shortly after she'd had a mastectomy. When I tried to assure her that she was being treated at an excellent hospital, she became even more angry and hung up. Two days later she called again, this time in tears, eager to tell me a story she had never related before, pleading with me to listen. I was totally unprepared for what followed.

She had been a victim of incest, repeatedly violated by her father from the time she was seven years old until she found the courage to run away when she was seventeen.

She married but purposely did not have children. She told no one about her father's incestuous acts and gave up all contact with her family.

After her husband died, she moved back to her hometown and, upon learning that her mother also had died, avoided contact with her father.

She didn't know that he had become a prominent benefactor of the hospital in which she had had her surgery, widely respected and loved by all.

When he learned she was there, he went to her. She was furious and told him to leave her alone. Instead, he spent hours with her at the hospital, causing her to become so hostile she was eventually sent to a psychiatrist, who also was an admirer of her father's.

When she had to undergo chemotherapy, her father drove her to the treatments, making his admirers admire him even more.

What they didn't know is that he once again was attacking his daughter, who, as she became increasingly weaker from her treatments, was unable to fend him off. He had put her in a position in which she needed his help and could do nothing to resist his sexual assault.

She was angry, hostile, and guilt-ridden, but it was a secret she could not divulge. Everyone thought it was cancer that had made her so hostile. No one knew it was really her father.

She was constantly told she was lucky to have a devoted father to care for her—instead of her having to care for him.

She told me that she would never reveal her secret to anyone and would not see a counselor. She did give me permission to pass on her story, though. Perhaps, indirectly, she wanted her friends and those treating her to know that her hostility, silence, and withdrawal had nothing to do with them.

If your efforts to reach out are rebuffed, don't conclude that the failure is yours. Other factors may be at work; there are some things you can't fix.

The stresses of illness and its treatment normally produce anger, fear, resentment, and depression in the patient. When these emotions are acted out, the target may be the medical staff. Inevitably, they are associated with the disease as much as with its control.

Patients don't mean to shoot the messenger, but bad news can provoke a shocked reaction. We can't will our illness away, but we can push away a nurse or snap at a technician.

Can a patient criticize the services received from the caregiving team, regardless of how ineffective the support may be, and not be ignored later for complaining?

Patients quickly learn that good behavior is rewarded. But what happens if a less-than-cooperative disposition and anger with the disease are allowed to surface around those directly responsible for the patient's needs? Will the patient then be ignored?

Will anger be met with anger, or will the doctor look for its cause and refer the patient to professional help as a way of helping the patient cope?

Will the patient seek the services of the hospital patient advocate? Does the patient know if the hospital has one?

Clearly there is a need for a middleman between the surgeon's table and the psychiatrist's couch. The best professionals try to make the climate as comfortable as possible and allow the patient to maintain his dignity. If patients are experiencing a lot of stress, ideally the health care team should deal with it by defining available resources—social worker, hospital chaplain, cancer therapist, support group.

Finally, all those involved must remember that what is human and forgivable in themselves is equally human and forgivable in those they treat.

10
Hope: Looking Forward

The ancient Greek writer Aesop told a tale of the great god Zeus, who once put all of life's blessings into a jar and entrusted them to the care of a mere mortal. The man, wanting to know what was inside, opened the jar, and everything flew out except for one thing—hope.

Aesop's moral: The only thing that promises man the recovery of blessings he has lost is hope.

Geo: It may be hard to think of a life-threatening illness as a prelude to a fuller life. But when the pain and fear subside, your experience will, if you let it, offer an opportunity to reach beyond yourself, to do things you've been putting off, to decide what's important to you, to make the rest of your life productive and happy.

Don't think about dying. Work at living. Your life can be more meaningful and enriching.

I was thirty-four years old when cancer and I discovered we had each other. By the grace of God and with the help of medical science, I am alive . . . but I've had to fight hard to stay alive.

I shudder to think of what would have happened if I had given up hope and had crawled into a corner waiting to die, then, after surviving for twenty years, realized that I had wasted a precious lifetime.

At the time of my diagnosis, I had no idea what the future would bring. No one does, of course. But, had I known how long the illness, surgeries, and recurrent problems would go on, I might have felt I'd been assigned an impossible task.

What if I'd received the following telegram?

Time: Noon, October 8, 1968

Place: My home, Chicago, Illinois

Telegram Arrives: Message: Within two days you will begin an ongoing battle with cancer. You will face surgery, radiation, recurrences, fear, anxiety, and repeated absences from home. You will have no recourse if you choose to live: BEGIN PREPARING IMMEDIATELY!

Your Mission Is: To survive, to accept, to persevere, to tend to your young children and properly raise them to adulthood. To continue to comfort your husband and keep your marriage strong.

You will experience adversity and hardship, loss of parents, family problems, and ongoing stress, but you must remain constant in your faith and be a source of strength and inspiration to others.

You will long for the carefree and cancer-free years, for the changes will be fast and furious . . . but you must never look back and question, "Why me?" Don't lose your sense of humor.

> If you follow all instructions care-
> fully, you'll emerge the victor and
> will indeed have accomplished "a
> mission impossible." Good luck!

Nobody receives such a telegram. Instead, we face new challenges one day at a time, and each day we are free to decide how we will respond.

Bud and I have met many, many people who confronted their problems by doing something positive:

Ned, a Call-PAC volunteer, wanted to coach Little League baseball when his sons were young, but he couldn't while receiving chemotherapy. He did, though, after he finished his treatments; and even though his own sons were no longer playing, he found satisfaction in coaching other kids whose fathers couldn't or were perhaps, as he had been, too ill.

Leann loved music and wanted to perform in a choir but couldn't make it to rehearsals. But after she was diagnosed and treated, she retired from her job and joined a group that sang at hospitals and schools.

Phyllis wanted to go to Hawaii but didn't get around to it until after she got sick. She finally went—in a wheelchair—with a close friend to help and enjoy it with her.

Ralph volunteered to drive other patients to their treatment after he completed his own.

Gerry became a volunteer guide at her local museum. Lenore opened a lingerie boutique when she encountered difficulty locating feminine garments following a mastectomy.

Shelley, a Hodgkin's disease patient, learned to fly an airplane. Why not? Flying might be dangerous, but no more so than cancer.

These patients chose to act positively to give joy and richness to their lives.

The most important thing to me was to preserve our love and cohesion as a family. Between the demands of my illness and Bud's erratic hours, it became a real challenge as the children grew older and had their own schedules to work around.

I recall with amusement the conversation with our dear editor, Susan Buntrock, when I proposed this book in May of 1987. I said I'd send some background materials when we returned from our vacation. She asked where we were going. "We're taking the children to Disney World." "How exciting," she said. "How old are the children?" I laughed and said, "Well, Kerry is twenty-one and Jim is twenty-four." It was a perfect example of how we have lived for many years, always having to postpone or change plans. We had to delay many trips for quite a while; but when we went, we *all* went, and we enjoyed our trips *immensely*.

Kerry was only two when I learned I had cancer. For as long as she can remember I've had an illness that has intruded rudely and continually into our lives.

I wasn't expected to survive, much less see Kerry and her older brother, Jim, through adolescence. But the surgeries, radiation, and pain were endured and perhaps made easier—or at least bearable—by my unflagging desire to see the children grow up.

After all, it seemed terribly unfair to have adopted two beautiful children and then not be around to raise them, so I made my arrangements with God, promising to endure without complaint whatever happened to me and to devote my life to helping others afflicted with illness in return for the gift of life.

The "arrangement" has worked but also has required monumental amounts of patience, compromise, and perseverance from all of us.

Far too many times our plans with the children were dashed at the last minute because I was hospitalized again. Bud was all too frequently beeped away when we needed him most. Civil rights marches, assassinations, riots, elections, and Olympic Games claimed equal time with my major operations.

Kerry was set to begin her first year of college out of state in 1985, but her plans were postponed because of my brain surgery.

She became my primary caregiver during the long and difficult recovery period. She attended a community college without complaint, continued working, drove me to my appointments, and helped in other ways. In appreciation of her sacrifices, I tried harder to do as much as I could for her.

Despite the difficulties, despite the many times our plans were changed by the necessities of Bud's job or the recurrence of my illness, we cherished the time we had together and drew strength from each other. And we made it through every rough period.

I didn't let statistics terrify me and prevent me from putting up the most powerful struggle of my life.

For twenty years we kept looking forward, enjoying the growth of our children, seeing them emerge as adults.

More anniversaries and birthdays were celebrated in hospital lobbies than at home, not in traditional ways or on exact dates, but they were, nevertheless, celebrated together.

Although my future was uncertain, we kept looking forward to the next important moment to remember. At times it's hard to believe I'm still leaving footprints after twenty operations. It's equally hard to believe I've been around for the important moments in my family's life: Jim's and Kerry's first dates, their graduations, our twenty-fifth wedding anniversary.

Each of those moments to remember came and went, and then, because of my remarkable recovery, we were on the threshold of another, Kerry's going away to college. I had to deal with her first extended period of time away from home. It was rough. I missed her terribly. But I was happy that she was finally able to pursue her education and thankful that my constant praying had given me more time.

Bud: Seeing our children through these important times has been an extra-special joy for us, but over the years we both have worried that Geo's illness was affecting the children in ways we could not see. Might they resent her? Might they leave home too soon? Might their lives be misdirected?

These are not unlike the concerns of all mothers and fathers, but our joy in seeing Jim and Kerry today, compassionate and caring after being harshly exposed to the realities of life at so young an age, is a reward reaped by just a few.

Despite the ups and downs that were jammed into our many years of living with cancer, we have managed to hang in there and forge what we feel is a beautiful family relationship. This is a solid plus and by itself has made our struggle worthwhile. It is a testament to Geo's strength and unyielding desire to preserve her role as wife and mother under very difficult circumstances.

In 1984, shortly after her brain surgery, the Lerner Newspapers in Chicago selected Geo as one of their "Citizen of the Year" honorees. She was uplifted by the honor, and it couldn't have come at a better time in her recovery. But she was very self-conscious about her puffed-up look, wobbly walk, and still slightly slurred speech.

She didn't want anyone to applaud because they felt sorry for her or thought that she wasn't going to be around much longer. She was determined to be there, though, to testify once more to the importance of the choices illness gives us. Here is part of what she said:

"I sometimes wonder why people receive awards simply for doing what needs to be done. But I am honored and grateful to have been selected Citizen of the Year, and I thank you.

"Happiness or unhappiness, I think, depends more upon the way we meet and deal with the events of our lives than on the nature of the events themselves. It is important to persevere because complaining doesn't change things, and it certainly doesn't solve your problems. One must make a commitment and carry on.

"But to tell you the truth, I think I would rather have fulfilled the childhood dream I had growing up in Iowa. I wanted to play the accordion, to sing, and to look like the late Kate Smith, 'Miss God Bless America,' whom I heard so often on the radio as a child in Council Bluffs. Instead, I became a 'sick' woman who persevered and won some awards.

"One of the things this honor means to me is that one can make a contribution even when life itself is under siege, and I'm happy someone has thought enough of my work to honor me with this award. Thank you very much."

Geo: That was six years ago, six years even more fulfilling than the ones preceding them.

Jim was married in April of 1990. His wife Ellen is beautiful, charming, and a lovely addition to our family. In fact, we became "instant" grandparents to Ellen's two small children, David and Leda.

I knew we had done something right when Jim came to talk with me before he asked Ellen to marry him. He told me he wanted a marriage as committed as ours, and did not consider divorce an option. Jim also said he had grown to love Ellen's children so much he wanted to adopt them after they were married. Bud and I considered Jim's comments the greatest compliment any parents could receive.

Kerry graduated from Purdue in December of 1989 and became engaged to Andrew Simerman, who graduated at the same time. They had met when she attended a reception at Andy's fraternity house in her first year at Purdue. He asked her to be his "little sister" then and four years later he asked her to be his wife. They were married in September of 1990.

It was as if a computer had matched Kerry and Andy.

He is very responsible, protective, gentle, and compassionate—the rare kind of person a father thinks is "good enough" to marry his daughter.

We couldn't be happier or more proud with the way things have worked out. We not only love the people our children have married, we love their families as well. We could not be more blessed.

At Kerry's wedding Bud proposed a toast and summed up our feelings, saying that when I first became ill the chances that I would be around for that happy day were not very good. But there I was, alive and well and very happy.

We made it!!!

Afterword

Geo: There were so many, many people we wanted to thank, friends and strangers alike, that it created a problem we didn't know how to solve. I went to church, where I prayed for guidance so often, and the thought came to me—why not a letter to God?—and my pen flowed.

Dear God:

It's hard to believe that more than seven thousand days have passed since I asked to make an "arrangement" with You. Through bad times and good times I have needed You, and You have always listened.

Each of us, I know, has a cross to bear, and I thank You for the special cross You gave to me, for it taught me that life is a special gift not to be wasted for a moment.

I am thankful that my cross came with someone special to help me bear it. My loving and devoted husband is unsurpassed in his faith, strength, and willingness to help me.

Our children, now twenty-two and twenty-five, carried an awesome burden of their own but have become beautiful, caring people. Thank You for allowing me to see them grow to adulthood.

I am keeping my promise to help other sick and distressed persons (I didn't realize there were so many) and, in doing so, have become happier and more productive than ever.

Thank You for helping me open doors that had been tightly sealed and give the people who treat us an understanding of our weaknesses and strengths; and for helping me give patients an understanding of the weaknesses and strengths of our caregivers . . . and of ourselves.

Bud and I have been counting the blessed kindnesses of our friends. There are so many that we'd need a three-volume compendium to acknowledge them individually. We haven't room for that, but we can express our gratitude for their good deeds.

We appreciate everything they have done, but most of all, we appreciate their prayers and gifts of faith. Holy oil from the Holy Land. A tree planted in Jerusalem. A cross fashioned from the wood of an olive tree. Prayers from several continents, from people of different races and different creeds, from young and old, healthy and ill.

We thank You for our friends and neighbors who found time to listen to us, to talk, to care and to help. We will always remember their unfaltering friendship and never-ending kindnesses.

For those who gave us sound advice and unwavering support; who drove me to my doctors or to church; who helped in our volunteer activities by typing, filing, answering letters; for those who took care of the children, and for their teachers and classmates who helped them maintain school activities.

For friends and strangers alike, whose encouragement helped us through rough days: for those who put up with my tears and mood swings; who came to my home or hospital room to help me look better when I most needed uplifting; who helped with car and household repairs when we couldn't afford them.

We remember the residents, nurses, aides, technicians, physical therapists, and support personnel who assisted in my care and the people in the St. Francis Hospital laundry room who searched through eighty thousand bed sheets and linens to find the cross I had forgotten to unpin from my own when my bed was changed.

We remember the support of volunteers and co-workers: American Cancer Society friends and staff; Call-PAC volunteers; our friends at the FBI who have remained close and who've helped in countless ways.

We appreciate Bud's superiors and colleagues, who had to work harder and longer when he was beside my hospital bed, and their families, for they also made sacrifices.

Thank You for the patients who have permitted us to tell their true stories under made-up names. They taught us much. We mourned for those who did not survive and intensified our efforts as they asked us to do.

For others' faith in our work: the newspaper, radio, and television stations that invited us to articulate the needs of patients; the groups that invited me to lecture; the many health care professionals who respected my role as patient advocate.

Bless You for sending the elderly Greek man I met at the radiation clinic. He told me about his boyhood friend, Nectarios, who became a priest, a bishop, and then the first twentieth-century saint canonized by the Greek Orthodox Church. He gave me a relic of Saint Nectarios and told me to pray to him for he was the patron saint of cancer patients.

And for sending those who helped me arrange an annual service of Holy Unction on the Feast Day of St.

Nectarios in which thousands have participated, seeking spiritual healing.

(And yes, Lord, thank You even for the lady who stole
my purse and disposed of everything except the relic,
left behind in her jail cell at my request. I kept my
promise not to press charges if she would return the
relic to me; she kept her promise, too.)

We remember our sisters, their families, our aunts
and uncles, our cousins and *koumbari* (godparents),
whose lives were affected by my long-term illness.

You know all their names and all whose deeds I may
have neglected to mention. I offer my thanks and ask
You to hold them closely to You.

Most of all, Dear God, I thank You for the gift of life.

Georgia
March 1988

However far we have gone, or how little, the greatest distance we have to travel is within ourselves.

Bud: We said at the beginning that this was a book
about survival, and we hope the things that helped us
will also help you.

We cannot be certain why Geo survived. Her health
has been assaulted repeatedly, and she pursues her
commitment with such dedication she often cannot
separate her roles and works until she is in a state of
near exhaustion. She sleeps only three or four hours
most nights, yet she works harder than most healthy
people and looks better than they do, too.

Was it her promise to God, the skills of her doctors,
the wonders of medical science, her own strength and
determination to confront problems rather than ignore
them, the large support base her warmth and openness
have brought her?

It's probably all of these, but whatever it is, we're not
going to analyze it. We're simply going to be grateful

and look forward to our fiftieth anniversary and other magic moments, such as becoming grandparents (not too soon, though).

Over the years, many people have expressed their admiration to me for giving Geo courage and strength, for helping her fight her illness and keeping her promise to help others, but I don't really deserve it.

Despite the relentless assault on her body and the unremitting pain she has endured, it really is Geo's strength that has pulled us through, Geo's courage that has sustained us both.

As we said, this book is about survival. But it's also about love.

It would have been easy for Geo to give up, but she cared so much for us that she never gave in, and under very difficult circumstances she has held our family together.

I love her!

One Thing More . . .

The time of diagnosis usually is so shocking and stressful and so much energy is dissipated by negative emotions that very little is left to pursue or even to consider all existing sources of information and support.

In this section we've tried to suggest sources that are immediately available, no matter where you live or what you want to know. The best way to prevent fear from overwhelming you and your family is to get instant and accurate information on the disease, where to find a doctor if you don't have one, and coping and support groups in your area.

To help you avoid a frantic and frustrating search, which often results in finding outdated or conflicting information, we suggest calling the two cancer organizations listed below. They can provide the most up-to-date information available relative to your own needs—anything from treatment centers to support groups closest to your home.

Any list of resources is incomplete the moment it is published because new ones are always being created. But the fact that a list can be made is a testament to the huge advances in this area since 1968, when our own search for information and help resulted in frustration and disappointment. At that time there were barely any support groups and little information about them.

Today, happily, many coping groups, some based on sites of cancer, are instantly available. You need only to pick up the telephone to learn what is available in your area of the country.

WHERE TO ASK—WHAT TO ASK

No matter what your question about cancer, the best way to start is with two toll-free phone calls:

The American Cancer Society (ACS) is a national voluntary health agency, funded by private donations.
1-800-ACS-2345

The National Cancer Institute (NCI) is a federally funded branch of the National Institutes of Health.
1-800-4-CANCER

These numbers are answered during normal business hours, and both organizations will send you printed material at *no charge*. Each information program has strengths and weaknesses; take the time to call *both*.

Before you call, though, think a bit about what you want to know. Information about cancer falls into these general categories:

1. Cause/Prevention—What steps can people take to reduce their risk? What are the known carcinogens (cancer-causing agents)? What is known about the cause(s) of a particular cancer?

2. Detection—This area covers screening programs for people without any symptoms, like the pap smear, the test for hidden blood in the stool, or the mammogram.

3. Diagnosis—What tests are used to diagnose cancer? What physical effects are involved? Do the procedures hurt? Do they carry any risks?

4. Sites—You may be interested in "everything" about a particular cancer—lung, breast, colon, etc. Be sure to ask about the primary site, i.e., where the cancer first developed.

5. Treatment—What is usually done to treat the cancer? Surgery? Radiation? Chemotherapy? A combination? If a particular treatment plan has been suggested or a particular drug proposed, ask about that. Ask where to buy a wig, a breast prosthesis, a bathing suit, etc., if you should need them.

Referral practices vary from state to state, so if you want a referral to another doctor or hospital, don't just ask for a name. Ask how a doctor (or hospital) gets on the referral list. What are the criteria?

6. Rehabilitation—What long-term effects of the cancer or its treatment might be expected? Will physical rehabilitation be needed?

7. Support services—What services are available in the community—support groups, counseling, financial aid, etc? (We have not attempted to list such groups in this book because the information changes constantly. The ACS is particularly helpful here because it uses computer-stored information that is updated often.)

When speaking with each organization, indicate the reason for your call and ask the questions you planned to ask. Some helpful concluding questions:

"Is there anything else you can think of that I need to know?"

"Is there any other organization with information that would be helpful to me?"

"If you cannot answer my question, do you know who can?"

Further Reading

After you have received information from the American Cancer Society and the National Cancer Institute, you may wish to go further. Libraries and bookstores can help. Remember, however, that books deal best in information that does not change quickly. They can provide good information on coping, but specific group references may be obsolete. Medical libraries are not always open to the public; even when they are, their material may be overly technical.

Check with your doctors for pamphlets they routinely give patients. Contact your hospital's social services department and department of pastoral care. They'll know about local support services and may be able to suggest reading that has been helpful to others in your particular situation.

Other Phone Lines

Information about toll-free phone services, whether for cancer or some other chronic or life-threatening illness, can be obtained from the 800 operator. Dial 1-800-555-1212. For example: If you're interested in breast cancer, the operator can tell you about the Y-ME Breast Cancer Support Group whose number is 1-800-221-2141.

Cancer Call-PAC, which operated within area code 312, closed its lines in 1987. When we began in 1973, nothing like it existed; since then, however, hospital-based support services have proliferated, and ACS has expanded its patient visiting programs. We are gratified that Call-PAC helped so many and that its existence prompted others to focus on the needs we identified. In fact, one of the founders of Y-ME was originally a Call-PAC volunteer.

PHYSICIAN DATA QUERY (PDQ)

PDQ, designed for doctors by the National Cancer Institute, contains (1) prognostic and treatment information of all the major cancers; (2) summaries of all the clinical trials supported directly by NCI, including detailed information on the objectives, patient entry criteria, treatment regimen, and current information about who is performing the trial and where it is being conducted; and (3) a physicians' directory containing the names, addresses, and telephone numbers of approximately ten thousand physicians who devote a major portion of their clinical practice to the treatment of cancer.

Who can use PDQ? Generally, physicians, hospitals, and health organizations. Since most people are interested in PDQ for the clinical trial information, their best bet is to ask their physician, who can either directly call up the information or ask the hospital medical librarian to do so.

The National Cancer Institute (via 1-800-4-CANCER) will provide you with PDQ data, but we suggest you then review the material with your physician.

Other Computer Databases

Your neighbor, the computer whiz, may tell you about other computer databases, like MEDLARS, MEDLINE, CANCERPROJ, CLINPROT, and CANCERLIT. Designed for biomedical professionals, they include research projects, abstracts of medical journals, and more. More accessible versions of information relevant to your needs are available elsewhere.

CLINICAL TRIALS

In cancer research, a clinical trial is a study conducted with cancer patients, usually to evaluate a new treatment. Each study is designed to answer scientific questions and to find new and better ways to help cancer patients. Through clinical trials, researchers learn which approaches are more effective than others.

The term *clinical trial* should not be confused with *latest* or *best treatment*. Until the trial has been completed, no one will know what, if any, benefits will be gained.

It is relatively easy to locate trials, but deciding whether to participate is not. The American Cancer Society, Illinois Division, Inc., offers these considerations:

Some Reasons Patients Find Trials Attractive:

1. Access to an experimental drug for which preliminary data is promising.
2. The benefit of close supervision by the investigator.
3. The satisfaction of helping in the accumulation of new knowledge that may result in improved treatment.

Some Reasons Patients Decline to Participate in Trials:

1. Additional testing will be required, such as blood tests, x-ray, CAT scans.
2. The treatment already available may prove to give better results than the procedure being investigated.
3. Clinical trials may produce unexpected side effects and/or disease that occurs later.

Questions to Assist in the Decision-Making Process:

1. Does the study compare different treatment plans? Does it compare one drug to a placebo? (A placebo is an inactive substance; thus the study compares

one drug to no drug.) Will you know what part of the study involves you?

2. What risks and benefits may be expected?
3. What tests will be required? How often?
4. How many outpatient trips to the site of the program will be necessary?
5. What costs (for example, medication, laboratory tests, transportation) are covered by the study?
6. What happens if you wish to withdraw from the study?

Before you decide, make sure all your questions have been answered and that you understand the answers.

HEALTH INSURANCE

Continuing Insurance After Employment (COBRA)

In 1985, Congress passed the Consolidated Omnibus Budget Reconciliation Act (COBRA).

Briefly, the act requires employer-sponsored group health plans, with certain exceptions, to provide employees and their dependents the opportunity to continue to participate in the employer-sponsored health benefits plan after their coverage would otherwise cease. (Employers not affected include the United States government, the District of Columbia, churches, and employers with fewer than twenty employees during the preceding year.)

Employers may require covered persons to pay for continued participation, which lasts from eighteen months to three years, depending on the status of the person entitled to coverage. *You must enroll in a COBRA plan within thirty days of job termination.* Therefore, if you anticipate a job change or termination and wish to take advantage of the options provided for under the act, be sure to see your personnel director either before you leave or within thirty days of leaving.

Insurance With a History of Cancer

Insurance companies are beginning to admit persons with a cancer history into group plans on a site-by-site basis, rather than automatically refusing anyone who has ever had a cancer diagnosis. In order to find these companies, consult an independent insurance agent or write to the National Underwriters Company, 420 E. 4th St., Cincinnati, OH 45202, and ask for the publication *Who Writes What in Life and Health Insurance.*

Comprehensive Health Insurance Policy (CHIP)

Some states have passed legislation to create, in effect, a high-risk pool for citizens who cannot otherwise obtain health insurance. Participants must prove they have been rejected by insurers for health reasons. Costs generally run 125 percent to 150 percent of standard fees. To find out if your state has such a plan, contact your state attorney general's office or the state Department of Insurance.

About the Authors

Georgia Photopulos is the triumphant survivor of nineteen cancer-related surgeries, 120 cobalt treatments, and a twentieth operation for a benign cyst on the brain. A pioneer in emotional support systems for cancer patients, she founded Cancer Call-PAC, a twenty-four-hour hotline for the American Cancer Society—the first such hotline in the nation. Georgia is a well-known speaker and syndicated columnist whose accomplishments have won her honors across the country, and she continues to bring hope and inspiration to others suffering from a life-threatening illness.

Bud Photopulos has achieved three decades of distinction in broadcast journalism with ABC Television News. Presently a writer, producer, and reporter at ABC News in Chicago, his reports have been featured on ABC's "Evening News" and "Good Morning America," on the Armed Forces Radio Network, and, through syndication, in many countries around the world.